Sharing Sadhana

Sharing Sadhana

Insights and Inspiration for a Personal Yoga Practice

Victoria Bailey

ROWMAN & LITTLEFIELD PUBLISHERS, INC.
Lanham • Boulder • New York • Toronto • Plymouth, UK

Published by Rowman & Littlefield Publishers, Inc.
A wholly owned subsidiary of The Rowman & Littlefield Publishing Group, Inc.
4501 Forbes Boulevard, Suite 200, Lanham, Maryland 20706
www.rowman.com

10 Thornbury Road, Plymouth PL6 7PP, United Kingdom

British Library Cataloguing in Publication Information Available

Library of Congress Cataloging-in-Publication Data

Bailey, Victoria.
Sharing sadhana : insights and inspiration for a personal yoga practice / by Victoria Bailey.
p. cm.
Includes bibliographical references and index.
ISBN 978-1-4422-1380-7 (cloth : alk. paper) -- ISBN 978-1-4422-1382-1 (electronic)
1. Healers--Biography. 2. Yoga--Therapeutic use. I. Title.
RZ407.B35 2012
613.7'046--dc23

2011052687

The paper used in this publication meets the minimum requirements of American National
Standard for Information Sciences Permanence of Paper for Printed Library Materials,
ANSI/NISO Z39.48-1992.

Printed in the United States of America

With a grateful love to Tim, Charles, Finn, and Alice

Contents

Acknowledgments

First, I would like to thank Suzanne I. Staszak-Silva, and the staff of Rowman & Littlefield for their faith, encouragement, and professionalism in all that they do. I would like to thank Susan Scott and Salima Stanley-Bhanji for their unconditional support and professional advice. I am truly blessed to call you both friends.

I would like to extend a sincere thank you to all the experientially insightful and confidently truthful yoga teachers and therapists who agreed to be interviewed for the purpose of this book, I will be forever grateful to you for sharing your stories. To the yoga teachers I have had, I am grateful daily for the knowledge you have shared, and if we lead by example, you have inspired in me a lifelong appreciation of sadhana.

Introduction

Chances are you have, have had, or are in the process of establishing or are hoping to create a personal daily yoga practice—a sadhana. A daily yoga practice, or sadhana, is carried out by yogis and yoginis throughout the world every day. A "Yoga in America" study released by *Yoga Journal* in 2008 reported that 15.8 million people in the United States practice yoga[1] while the North American Studio Alliance website estimates the number is higher at potentially 30 million practitioners in the states.[2] Through all these statistics though, one point remains; these people, that is, perhaps you and I, *practice* yoga and they (we) are considered to be yoga *students*.

Within Western culture, our knowledge of yoga and yoga practices has been somewhat shaped by lessons and insights provided and shared by often well-known yoga teachers. The *Yoga Journal* study also reported that the yoga industry in the United States alone generates $5.7 billion a year[3] through yoga classes, media and products. Yet throughout all the yoga courses I have completed, the one constant and consistent message from all teachers has been this: "You have to maintain your own daily practice— honor your sadhana."

However, the same teachers have not elaborated on or spoken to how they came to develop their own sadhana. They did not share in detail why they picked one tradition of yoga over another or how they may have amended aspects of that tradition over their years of practice to suit their needs. They either have not had the opportunity to offer guidance or have offered conflicting guidance on how to best find the most suitable personal practice. They also did not share information about why they decided to devise a very individualistic yoga practice that they change from day to day or season to season or advise how to best adapt your own sadhana throughout your own life and yoga journey.

I don't think these teachers were necessarily unwilling to share their experience. I think it is more that students can be (and I certainly was) too intimidated to ask their teachers about their respective individual sadhana; it is a *personal* practice. In these teachers' defence, who I am sure most likely would not want to intimidate their students in anyway, they are usually presenting a particular workshop or class to inform students about a specific tradition or application of yoga. Although instructors might offer their own perspective on an aspect of yoga, they aren't usually presenting information specifically about themselves.

The idea for *Sharing Sadhana* came to me while practicing yoga (it really did). Finding and committing yourself to a particular yoga tradition's daily discipline or finding the confidence and dedication to create your own yoga practice can be challenging to new yoga students, while it can become an essential part of everyday to people with an established practice. I struggled to cultivate my own sadhana, but eventually, with a bit of determination, a lot of practice and in spite of ill-timed waves and instances of self-doubt, illness, responsibilities, and daily time constraints, it came. However, it was accompanied by the epiphany that if I complete my personal practice, I feel great. Not to seem negative, but the flip side to this equation is that when I do not complete it, I do not feel as great. (I somehow missed that caveat on my yoga class waiver).

The main focus of creating *Sharing Sadhana* was to consult with prominent and experienced yoga teachers and therapists in the Western yoga world and to offer a means for these experienced practitioners to share their own development of sadhana, to provide insights into their own personal yoga journey as well as sadhana guidance and inspiration to new and seasoned yoga practitioners. For the sake of conciseness and clarity the content of the conversations was edited into a more readable format for the purpose of this book.

In the chapters of this book, I take the word sadhana to mean what the individuals interviewed explain it means to them. When I began my yoga teacher training, the first yoga instructors I had referred to sadhana as both our path *and* our daily practice. When I speak of sadhana in this book that is the meaning I adhere to. However, on a daily basis in my own North American suburban home, neither term is used—yoga is typically referred to in the possessive sense, for example, "Did you do *your* yoga this morning?" "Leave Mom alone; she's doing *her* yoga." "Mom, are you still doing *your* yoga?" "I'm going to do *my* yoga; if you need anything, ask Dad." Do I make lifestyle choices on a daily and bigger-picture basis that will affect my sadhana? Yes, but the reverse is also true. I feel my personal practice has blossomed and changed the way I live my life and respond to events and non-events alike on my own path for the better, and it helps guide me in a positive way.

Yoga was historically taught by, and practiced by men. Yet according to the 2008 "Yoga in America" study, by far the majority of yoga practitioners in North America are women—some 72.2 percent.[4] In *Sharing Sadhana*, I have purposely interviewed and gained perspectives from both men and women not because I think yoga should be viewed through a gender lens but rather with the aim of promoting balance within the scope of the included teachers. I also decided to interview teachers who sought out and/or discovered and who are dedicated to a particular school or tradition of yoga and, alternatively, those who, having completed much in the way of personal practice and yoga training, have gleaned influence from many sources, blended that into a yogic application for themselves, and gone on to share the strategies and tactics of their yoga practice with others.

The chapters of this book are focussed on teachers who are considered to be North American, that is, yogis and yoginis who are prominent within the Western yoga field. They may have visited or lived in India and/or many other places around the globe, but ultimately they are from or have settled in North America and are currently shaping yoga for Western practitioners through workshops, teacher trainings, retreats, CDs, DVDs, books, podcasts, articles, and so on. Perhaps once too they were just your "average Joe" or your "average Joanne" living in a rural area, in middle-class suburbia, or in an urban high-rise apartment, yet something occurred in their lives that led them to yoga within their North American existence, and they managed or actively sought to carve out a sadhana for themselves.

The first question I asked of all the yoga practitioners interviewed was, "What does sadhana mean to you?" and the conversation and resulting chapter and book evolved from there. Rabindranath Tagore, in *Sadhana: The Realization of Life*, states, "It is best for the commerce of the spirit that people differently situated should bring their different products into the market of humanity, each of which is complementary and necessary to the others,"[5] and that in essence is the spirit of this text: sharing.

My goal was not to compare, prescribe, or dictate how a sadhana should look or be expressed or experienced in any way. It is simply to share information about individual experiences of personal yoga practice—to provide insights and inspiration that could perhaps illuminate what is already inside of you, and encourage all of us to take ownership of our sadhana with truth and compassion.

I have been questioned by friends about the use of the word sadhana in the title. I don't think yoga is going to disappear from our cultural realm anytime soon and I think it can be advantageous to at least become comfortable or at ease with it. Similar to visiting a foreign language–speaking country, I wouldn't typically spend years studying for a BA (Hons) degree in that language before I plan my trip. But it would be helpful to learn a few of the key terms that will help me communicate with the people I come into contact with on that journey and help enrich my whole experience of that culture I am exploring.

Language has a vibration and ultimately, on this issue, I refer to my son, who pointed out to me one day, "You know that om thing you say. Om is what everyone in the world says when they don't know what to say." Sadhana helps us to be a little more mindful in those moments. Namaste.

NOTES

1. "Yoga Journal Releases 2008 'Yoga in America' Market Study," *Yoga Journal*, press release, http://www.yogajournal.com/advertise/press_releases/10, February 26, 2008.
2. "A Growing Profession: 70,000 Yoga Teachers Estimated by NAMASTA," North American Studio Alliance, http://www.namasta.com/pressresources.php, April 12, 2005.
3. "Yoga Journal Releases 2008 'Yoga in America' Market Study,"
4. "Yoga Journal Releases 2008 'Yoga in America' Market Study,"
5. Rabindranath Tagore, *Sadhana: The Realization of Life* (Minneapolis: Filiquarian Publishing, 2006), 14.

Chapter One

Paul Grilley

Paul Grilley is responsible for creating the *Anatomy for Yoga* DVD, the *Chakra Theory and Meditation* DVD, and the *Yin Yoga* practice DVD and book, and he provides related international teacher training programs and workshops. His comprehensive approach to yoga blends his knowledge of anatomy and physical movement with Eastern philosophy and yoga principles.

Thus, we have a paradox: Paul Grilley is a very self-aware and mindful individual who makes conscious choices about whether to include aspects of spirituality in his classes, DVDs, books, teacher trainings, and workshops. Paul's *Yin Yoga* trainings and supporting materials have led to him often becoming associated with the importance of understanding anatomy as a yoga teacher and practitioner. However, his advanced level of teacher training and more recent *Chakra Theory and Meditation* DVD and related training are of a more spiritual inclination and may even surprise some people who are used to associating Paul Grilley with the more anatomical attributes of yoga. As Paul himself declares, "Sometimes people are shocked at the level of learning and literature and philosophy that I have behind me because I don't bring it forward in a yoga class."

Paul Grilley was the first interview I scheduled and completed for this book. Related to this point, I will unashamedly reveal that I'm a bit of a control freak, if you can actually be described as only partially being of that mind-set. One of the reasons I was attracted to my now husband was that he is one of the few people I have met with a tighter itinerary and sturdier organizational skills than myself. I joked that he was "just like me, except 10 percent more so." To qualify being held in this regard by me, he has, in his past, completed military training and used to guard the Canadian Governor General's home in Ottawa; the man's shoes are *always* polished.

For this, my first interview, I had three methods of recording our conversation prepared, questions listed and printed, and backup pens. I had requested that my overseas relatives not call and had plans of containment for the family cat. However, I hadn't planned on karma—my karma. Maybe inadvertently it was Paul's fault; perhaps his heightened spiritual energy kicked my karma into gear. Whether Mr. Grilley was to blame or not, karma was at play. I was so busy being organized that I forgot to be organized. When Paul called through on the computer, I was peeling mushrooms in the kitchen, not professionally sitting in prepared expectation. Having skipped breakfast and just returned from a rather sweat-inducing yoga class, I had my mind-set on eating, showering, and meditating, all in time for locking the cat in the laundry room before what I *thought* was the scheduled time for our interview. As it happened, I mixed up the time zones.

"Hi there, I called you by accident. I was just trying to get set up," greeted Paul when I pushed the answer button. I couldn't very well push the decline button, could I? Although it was tempting, I hadn't even brushed my hair. The karma continued: "Would you like to call back?" I asked hopefully. I was very grateful then—and still am—for Paul taking the time out of his schedule for the interview and the wonderful insights that he was open to sharing, but I wanted to look my professional yoga teacher/writer person best. Instead, my being caught unawares had resulted in what I can only describe as a feeling that even my eyelids were spontaneously and uncontrollably sweating. I have only ever experienced a worse incident of nervous-induced sweating once before, and that was the day I met my now in-laws for the first time. Thankfully, the interview with Paul did not bring about a relentless sweating in my palms (apparently only my mother-in-law, who is actually, it turns out, very sweet, can do that)."No we're good, I'm ready," he replied. I smiled. Inside I was aagghhhhing. Yes, that is a word because it was what I was doing at that very moment, albeit internally, while I gathered together notebooks, pens, and recording devices.

Yet Paul's manner put me at ease right away, the calmness of his presence filling my office no doubt in some way fueled by the deep, internally focused meditation Paul completes as part of his sadhana with his wife Suzee each day. "We meditate every day, and there is a slight breadth of options available to the meditation. There are various ways that we draw our energies inward to the spine that does vary from week to week, month to month. The meditation is daily; the precise, specific technique does vary somewhat. I play basketball every day as a professional and every team I play against is different, but my goal is the same: beat this guy and put the ball in the hoop. However, one day I need to go over him, the next day around him, the next day I need to pass the ball to my teammate—the goal is the same every day. It isn't like there's one technique, and I do it six times, and then I change. To me that is a dead sadhana."

Life within sadhana and sadhana within life seems key to Paul and indisputably linked. When Paul first came to understand the term sadhana, it didn't seem unfathomably grueling or unattainable. Instead, it offered a positive objective. As Paul explains, "It didn't feel overwhelming, it felt like it gave a purpose and a meaning to life, which I think is about as big a thing as you can say about anything. It was instantly tied in with the notion that there is a possibility of spiritual advancement."

Paul discovered this knowledge of spiritual purpose through study: both self-study and the study of philosophical texts. "I was interested in human potential, and I dabbled in things in early high school like training your memory. I'd read about how people under hypnosis could do extraordinary things. So as I was interested in the idea of human potential I found college frustrating because it didn't talk directly to those things. I came home after a disappointing couple of years of college and made a list of things that I was actually interested in, none of which were academic courses, like mind over matter, hypnosis, memory training, all those things, and all of them were on the outside of academic respectability.

"I went to the only sort of 'off the wall' guy in our town who I could think of who was a chiropractor thinking, 'Well, he might have a view into things that are not ordinary.' He made a list of three books for me, two of which were theosophical books and one was *Autobiography of a Yogi*. It just turned out that the theosophical books were difficult to get; this was before the Internet and Amazon. The first and easiest book to acquire was Yogananda's *Autobiography of a Yogi*. I literally stayed up nights reading that book. I read every footnote—everything in that book I digested. It was an extraordinary introduction to a different way of seeing the world and seeing life. I went from having an interest in 'What is the human potential?' to 'Oh my God, the human potential is infinitely greater than I was thinking.' I would have been content to learn powers of mind over body or how to do self-hypnosis to train yourself to do different things, but then you start reading, 'No, your goal as a human being is to unify with God and the infinite.' It stretched my boundaries way beyond my original inclination."

Paul considers reading *Autobiography of a Yogi* a pivotal moment in his life, one that ultimately led him onto the personal and professional path he is on today. The revealing of a perception of the world to which he had so far not been exposed was both astonishing and impactful. "I read that book when I was nineteen years old and the very idea that there are altered states of consciousness, that there are exalted states of spirituality, and that there are systematic techniques and pathways by which to achieve those insights was completely new to me. The notion that you could aspire to a spiritual state and that there were many long traditions about what to do to get there was a shocking revelation that no one had mentioned to me before; I was sort of stunned. It's like coming across a view of the world that seems the most important thing in the world, and no one had talked about it previous to me reading that book. It felt like, 'Did I miss a class in high school where this stuff was discussed?' It isn't like I had this idea before that there are exalted spiritual states but didn't know how to get there. I had no idea that there *were* exalted spiritual states. I was raised in a fairly religious disinterested family, so I was taken aback and wowed by a complete worldview that I had no idea previously existed."

Through study and commitment, Paul is now at a place where sadhana means something to him far more than time spent on a mat or meditating. "To me sadhana implies discipline, meaning things that you might not do because we all have inertia against changing habits. It's easier to skip meditation, it is easier to not do certain things, it is easier to read books that are fluff than to try to crack your head open against something that is deeper and harder to understand. Every one of those steps takes a willful effort, and I think that that is sadhana. In the broader context, I think if sadhana is innately behind everything you do in your life and you remind yourself constantly 'My goal is to progress spiritually,' then it influences everything that you do."

While Paul may not refer to the term of sadhana on a daily basis, he does refer to the intention of his sadhana itself. "I share my sadhana with my wife Suzee. We both innately understand the term, we just don't sit around and say, 'How was your sadhana?' We say things like 'How was meditation for you this morning?' and we are in constant discussion with each other about how we behave particularly with other people throughout the day. We constantly review our interactions with other people, and we do it with an idea of 'Did we behave in a way that was in accordance with our spiritual ideals?' We act and behave in a way that is sadhana; we just don't use the term."

For Paul, sadhana is linked to choices you make in life. "The broader context of sadhana, to me, means your goal in life is spiritual. Sometimes frequently this means it's at odds with advancing yourself in name, fame, and money, and so you will make decisions sometimes, not always, that are not in your best professional interest, but you determine they are in your best spiritual interest. I think if you make decisions like that, you're doing that because you have an overarching philosophical view of the world, and if it influences your decisions in any way, then I think that you're practicing sadhana. Otherwise, you just follow the money or you take anyone's advice who comes along. Everyone's got advice for you on how to live your life."

That doesn't mean Paul has found that to feel successful in a spiritual life, you need to *not* be successful in a more traditional Western way. "I don't believe that spirituality is contradictory to success. There's nothing wrong with being famous, there's nothing wrong with being successful. I do not think that these are contradictory things, but sometimes the best thing to do spiritually might not be *the* best thing to do financially. Sometimes they'll converge. I think that is a definition of sadhana: where every decision you make is somehow framed or considered relative to sadhana because otherwise we wouldn't consider them."

However ingrained sadhana is in Paul's life, there was a conscious effort to cultivate and realize his personal practice through the application of self-discipline. As he explains, "In spite of having a hatha yoga practice from the beginning, it was not easy for me to sit. When I found a way to sit and be comfortable, I thought, 'Wow, this is amazing.' There have been many, many little things like that that knock away internal hindrances that you're not always aware are there. For the first eight to ten years, I was trying to get my house in order in terms of 'What do I do externally, and when do I legitimately carve out time in my day that's not professionally or family oriented and sit down and do my practice?' I think that was the biggest struggle."

However, literature helped provide Paul with sadhana guidance. "I think much in the beginning was reading and rereading inspirational materials about what you should do with your life. I don't think that's a waste of time. I think it's a necessary thing to do, but thank God I'm at a place now where I don't need to read material to inspire me to sit and do my practice; the practice itself is rewarding. I was feeding my mind and feeding my conceptions of what is the best way to live your life, but I was twenty-something, I was trying to find a job, trying to earn a living, trying to find a mate. There's a lot going on in your life, and so it took me a long time to get from 'This is what you should be doing' to 'Hey, I'm doing it.' "

When you are redefining yourself in that way, sometimes, not always, the change can be a struggle both for yourself and for others. Myself and other people I know who have chosen a more spiritual or more self-aware yogic path are sometimes criticized and encouraged to slip back into old habits by both casual acquaintances and people they love. My personal "favorite" is the friend who tells me over and over, "You're boring now." I know the life I have led and lead, and it's truly anything but boring. There was a point early on in my yoga studies, though, where get-togethers and invitations to events made me anxious, and I would obsess on points such as, "How will people react if I don't drink alcohol with them because I want to get up early tomorrow and do my yoga practice?"

Paul can relate to this kind of situation but encourages staying true to yourself and your lifestyle choices. "Meditation is the ultimate, iconic effort to control our minds and our reactions, but we can make an effort to control our mind and our reactions every instant of our life. If you decide 'I'm going to go out with my friends and show them that I'm a normal, beer-drinking, backslapping guy just like them,' that's okay. But if you go out and party like that and do some things that are innately against what you believe, for example, flirting with women when you're a married man or doing drugs when you really don't do drugs, then you've abandoned your sadhana. But if you can go out and do that and be true to your moral convictions you're still involved in your sadhana. Is it the ultimate sitting down and controlling your mind? No, because you're distracted by a hundred different things, but it's not an abandoning of your sadhana to not do meditation. It's an abandoning of your sadhana if you get up and go do something other than meditate, then you just throw out the window all considerations of what your broader purpose in life is."

Paul's studies led to him joining Paramahansa Yogananda's Self-Realization Fellowship, followed by a gradual migration toward the teachings of Dr. Hiroshi Motoyama. Although, there was more of a combining component to that progression, as Paul explains. "Dr. Motoyama's teachings are, in my mind, completely compatible with Yogananda's teachings, but part and parcel of Dr. Motoyama's teachings are everybody's different, everybody's karma is different, everyone's energetic body is different. Though the principles are the same, the specific techniques and schedules and practices and environments in which they are practiced are going to vary. You've got to keep your eye on the prize. When a certain set of techniques and practices are no longer producing results for you that are desirable, then you have to have the courage to change."

Although it seems for Paul that his spirituality, philosophy, and lifestyle are certainly intertwined, with sadhana being an expression and an affirmation of that, he believes that we are suited to change. However, change in our lives can at times be difficult both for ourselves and for others. As Paul explains, "One of the conflicts that I had with the Self-Realization Fellowship was a constant haranguing of me about how hatha yoga is not the true spiritual path, hatha yoga is going to seduce you away from the spiritual path, hatha yoga is going to strengthen your ego. I would hear that all the time. Yet Yogananda taught hatha yoga to his disciples and demonstrated hatha yoga postures. Somehow in the modern interpretation that's been forgotten, and every time I would talk to someone in my sangha, my group of people, and say, 'I teach hatha yoga,' they would respond, 'Oh, really? Is that what you do? You need to be careful with that.' I could not buy into what those people were telling me my religion was saying about my profession. I don't think there was a spiritual cabal and everyone was plotting to undermine me, but this is what the circumstances of my life brought me to confront."

Through working through this sense of conflict, Paul's sadhana continued to evolve and began to take a different direction. "I slowly made my way out of the guru/disciple paradigm and into a more Western egalitarian academic paradigm, which, for all of its faults, I think is a safer way to share and create a sangha on spiritual ideas."

In terms of seeking that guidance for your own spiritual path, Paul advises letting your own requirements as a student determine your method of learning. "I think that different human beings have different capacities and tendencies. Some people hate school, hate classrooms, hate groups, and study better on their own. Other people love school, love classrooms, love groups, and feel lonely by themselves."

Paul also recommends letting apt literature continue to inform your practice. "Constantly reading works that people wrote who have preceded us in these endeavors is the smartest thing you can possibly do."

Though Paul advises being mindful of what you might choose to read. "Patanjali put the word 'swadhyaya' in his list of niyamas as an important thing. The mind needs to eat, you need to feed it. You can either pick junk food from TV and newspapers and inane casual conversation, or you can feed it little hard facts to chew on: spiritual phrases, spiritual books, poetry pointing to a higher ideal. If that's all you feed your mind for years and years and years, hopefully there's going to come a day when there isn't much room in your mind for the other stuff, and that's going to be a good day."

Yet Paul believes that you need to ensure your practice does not become so studied, structured and dogmatic that it becomes mindless routine. "All of the techniques, all of the prayers, all of the efforts are meant to expose us to altered states of consciousness that eventually will be our natural states of consciousness. Our goal is not to do as many pranayamas in this lifetime as we can. The goal for this life is not to see how many hours we can sit. The goal in this life is to achieve an exalted awareness of the presence of God in all things. Techniques are simply suggested ways to get there. In the end it's not about the technique, it's about a heartfelt awareness of God's presence everywhere at all times. If we become successful in our lives, all it will take is a turn of our thoughts, a turn of our mind, a whispered prayer, a silent affirmation, and we will move ourselves into that exalted state that took years to achieve the first time, but the second time was easier, the third time was easier, and the tenth time was even easier."

Whether that exalted state for you is a connection with God, Buddha, Mother Nature, Gaia, Jesus, energy, the universe, nature, yourself or a connection to something indescribable, Paul explains that we ultimately experience a paradox: the outside world will become clearer when we look inside. "It's innately appealing to me that the search for God has to be inside you. Is there a reflection of God in the outer world? Yes, of course, but I know people who all their life have their eyes and ears open to the outer world, and it doesn't lead them to spirituality. Whereas I do *not* think that the opposite is true. I do *not* think a wide-awake, conscious effort to cultivate healing and sensation inside of you is *not* going to open up spiritual doors."

Perhaps, though, more appropriately, rather than a paradox, this outlook is essentially yin and yang exemplified by Paul himself. The conscious time and effort Paul has strived to and continues to put into his personal practice is reflected back as a practical personal compassion, even if sometimes that is simply expressed as kind understanding toward people who are peeling mushrooms in their kitchen when their conscious efforts would be better focused elsewhere.

Chapter Two

Wade Imre Morissette

From a young age Wade Imre Morissette was drawn to music and physical movement that nurtured a spiritual connection and this inclination eventually led him to yoga. He became a certified yoga teacher and, inspired by a trip to India, began to integrate his love for music and yoga through practicing mantra, chanting, and kirtan, now a key element of his yoga teachings. Wade has created numerous music and chant recordings for yoga, including the CDs *Yoga Music Flows* (vols. 1 and 2), *Strong as Diamonds*, *Sargam Scales of Music*, and *Maha Moha—The Great Delusion*. He is also the author of *Transformative Yoga: 5 Keys to Unlocking Inner Bliss*.

The day that I was scheduled to interview Wade, there was not a lot of joy in my mind, mostly a building sense of angst for any one of the typical reasons anyone ever has that feeling and I was longing to practice yoga. I dropped my kids off and ran a few errands, and while in my local pharmacy I began chatting to one of the staff there. She had recently started coming to a studio where I teach, and we recognized each other. Originally from India, the lady and I started talking about yoga, and she explained that as a child she didn't practice asana but would join the adults in her family in a daily practice of chanting, mantra, and prayer. With a melancholy tone, she lamented, "I just didn't appreciate it for what it was at the time, and although yoga classes here are refreshing and relaxing, I miss that part of it."

Although the store is a kilometer or less from my home, I felt I wanted to run to my mat, the synchronicity of our conversation and my angst propelling me there, and simply cling to it. Instead, I practiced, creating the grounding sensation that I needed. Feelings of anxiety lingered all morning, but being somewhat subdued by my own yoga practice, I could watch it from a distance, waiting for the cloud to lift—that is, until I spoke to Wade Imre Morissette. He has three names. If I had to choose three words to describe him, they would be "joy," "joy," and "more joy." You can hear it in his voice and it resonates through his words and manner, his being. Apparently the joy he expresses also causes predatory feelings of anxiety to retreat.

For Wade, joy seems inherently linked with sound and he has observed that the incorporation of mantra and music into yoga practice is becoming more popular in the Western yoga world. As Wade explains, "The kirtan movement, chanting in groups and the repetition of mantra in meditation, is definitely widespread and popular right now, and I think it's because it is so tangible. Some people can't sit silently; it's impossible for certain people. The music is universal. Everyone can connect to music, it breaks down all barriers, and then you have the mantra aspect bringing them together, so you have enjoyment. Enjoyment is a big word for me; in enjoyment there is no rigidity. The music breaks down the barriers, and the mantra involves such an amazing language, and the practice of the meditation with these mantras is a great combination."

As a result, Wade is comfortable with Sanskrit terminology when it comes to practice. "I like the word sadhana, it works for me. I think sadhana is any type of practice that helps you connect with your essence and helps you meditate and focus your mind and connect to your deeper energy. Sadhana is definitely a discipline too; there's regularity to it. It's a regular practice that helps you connect within."

A creative and accomplished artist in his own right, Wade is also the twin brother of musician Alanis Morissette and not surprisingly, music plays an important part in his practice. "Music is so important to me. I can be creative with playlists and practicing with them. Music is probably at the forefront of what inspires me to practice."

For Wade it seems that sound in language, music, and mantra is unequivocally unified with joy and thus yoga in life, each one motivating and inspiring the other. "Joy is definitely crucial, and I always say to people, 'I'm an artist trapped in the yoga world,' which isn't necessarily a bad place to be trapped in. The sadhana, the yoga, incredibly inspires creativity and imagination. My sadhana is almost a vehicle to allow me to be in better creation and expression as an artist. Whenever I am in sadhana, I'm always inspired creatively on some level."

Humans are innately musical, and mantra and music, whether live or recorded, can help most of us in invoking a sense of inward focus or a change in mood or in bringing mindfulness into whatever we do, including sadhana. In the same way, Wade finds that practicing yoga alone or participating in a group yoga class can shape the energy of a practice. As he explains, "I definitely think group classes and a private personal practice are both incredibly beneficial. I think the key is that you are *practicing* whatever it is. Sometimes being in groups helps inspire you when you're feeling not so inspired, and so I do believe in the importance of group energy to lift spirit if you need it, but I also think personal private practice is important so that you can really focus with the mind without all the distractions of the people around you. There's a time and place for both; I'd almost recommend practicing both."

Wade was already practicing yoga regularly when he became aware of the Sanskrit term sadhana. Although Wade did make a conscious shift toward committing himself to a path of discovery in his late teen years, on reflection he thinks his sadhana existed before that time. "When I was young, I was in competitive swimming, and I didn't realize until I was older that that was a form of meditation, and that was the beginning of my sadhana almost. All you can hear when you swim is your breath, and so I would say my sadhana started even much earlier, but it wasn't defined as sadhana at that point for me—it was defined as swimming."

Yet this natural sense of sadhana helped direct Wade toward a more mindful path. "At eighteen, something shifted, and I realized that my shift was to live toward truth in whatever way that was. That's why I was so pulled to Eastern mysticism and all the Eastern philosophies essentially, including yoga and meditation. It was definitely a progression, a shift, but there was no defining sadhana point. It's been so changing and malleable. I know it's with me when I'm feeling connected and inspired, and then I know it's not with me when I'm feeling disconnected or in the darkness. It's the perfect compass and gauge for me to know when I'm connected or not."

Not to exhaust the musical puns or analogies, but I suppose that at times in life, slow, soft music fits and that at other times something more uplifting is in order. It's about what's right in the moment, just like sadhana, that makes it effective. Wade explains, "My practice means many things at different times. Sometimes it's fatherhood, sometimes it's being in my community, and sometimes it's being in headstand. I'm going to attempt to do an ironman in Brazil in 2013, and there's a lot of cardiovascular exercise involved, yet there are so many ways you can practice on focusing the mind. I like to keep my practice varied and eclectic to keep the entertainment factor high. You don't want your practice to ever get stagnant or become a chore or a task."

While Wade has amended his personal practice over the years to suit his needs, his experience of it has also changed as he has matured. "In my twenties my practice was very asana based. In my early thirties it was very meditation and mantra based. Now I'm getting back into the physicality of the enjoyment of movement and vinyasa and poses; it's like a wave. In training for this triathlon I know how essential the yoga asana practice will be in terms of maintaining the suppleness so there'll be less injury."

Wade has found that as he grows older and changes, so too how he responds to practice also changes. "There's a maturity as you get older where so much more happens energetically and with the mind in the poses versus

when you're in your twenties and you're eager and you're looking to challenge yourself and go deeper into poses. For me now, there's more of an
aspect of the mind, and I use mantra regularly as I practice, so it's becoming
more and more enjoyable as I mature."

However, incorporating movement in to practice remains key for Wade.
"What's important for me is movement; mindful movement. Having the
meditation within the movement is why I'm so attracted to mantra because
you can bring mantra into movement, or you can make it meditation. Those
are my two main compasses for what I offer when I travel and teach, and
what I believe in and what I practice myself. Those are the two main components: meditation and movement and then music, obviously, for enjoyment."

Wade's practice is rooted in checking in with himself and letting his
sadhana naturally evolve from there. "In Tantra philosophy it's shakti first,
then to shiva, meaning laying the foundation of listening and softening first,
and then there will be spontaneous action. I'm really trying to embody that in
my practice as well as when I teach. It's all about knowing that there's an
incredible amount of power at the end of an incredible softening."

Although he appreciates having such an ability to connect inside and find
and cultivate joy, Wade still believes in the importance of sadhana guidance.
"I think it's very important to have guidance and to never stop having guidance. I still have a lot of connections to my teachers that I reach out to, and I
think that's very important. Whether it has to be one person for your whole
life or you have a lot of different influences and people guiding you as you
evolve, it's very individual. Each person is going to have to figure out what
that looks like for them and what they need and where they are. Finding that
is so individualistic. What is common between everyone, whether you are at
beginner level or advanced, is that whoever is guiding you, whoever is inspiring you, or empowering you, if those qualities are present, if this is
happening, then have a hundred teachers or have one."

Wade believes that this inner and external guidance will serve you well
even when your sadhana seems unrewarding. "Pattabhi Jois had the saying,
'Do your practice, and all is coming.' I misconstrued that with a Western
mind to mean that if I didn't do my practice, all was going. Make sure there
is always joy within when you're practicing your sadhana. That's why I think
it has to change so quickly for some people because there is so much external
change in some people's lives. If they can get the basic tools and the knowledge and take that knowledge and bend it as their life takes twists and turns, I
think that is important."

Linking an appreciation to every moment we might experience both on
and off the mat, Wade explains, "In Tantra philosophy everything is an
experiment, and in that experiment we gather life experience and informa-

tion. I think in consciousness there is no regret. In consciousness there's a huge gratitude for every moment and experience, whether it be incredibly dark or incredibly light or anything in between."

Yet Wade emphasizes that it's always ultimately about balance. "What I'm trying to do is structure my lifestyle so I can be in quality time with my children and at the same time let my practice support that presence. That's the ultimate goal right now, making sure there is that balance between the two. Obviously there are moments when you're going to have to put all sadhana aside and step up and focus some more time on your child. It's ever changing, but a balance of both is the goal."

Sometimes, perhaps, there is a fine line between allowing your sadhana to become a mindful choice of taking your focus away from your mat and letting it be expressed as time spent with family or in your community and alternatively allowing a tamasic influence, that is, a force of sluggish inaction, imbalance you. Wade finds that having gentle lifestyle props of discipline in the form of a routine space and/or time for your sadhana can prove greatly beneficial. "Consistency in space and time is, for me, hugely important. For a lot of people, that familiarity means less thinking, and in familiarity you can soften your armor a little bit more. If a time doesn't work, soften in that moment as well, as far as saying, 'Well, now I need to change it or redefine it or change my perception of it.'

"It's like you have a blueprint and you work around that blueprint. My blueprint is sixty to ninety minutes of movement-based asana. It's very important for me physically right now to keep that physical asana happening on a daily basis. It's important so I don't have injuries. I think it will always change, but I believe that movement is important. Whether you are moving incredibly slowly or whether you're doing deep vinyasa movement between poses and postures, it's the same: the movement is the healing."

Wade also observes that your flow of breath can help guide your practice. "The premise for the practice is: is your breath easeful or not? The movement is the vehicle for the prana."

Yet he acknowledges that how your sadhana might look will change. "Sadhana will always have a different meaning to you. Sometimes it's really close, and sometimes you think about what you need to do in your life to bring it back. We all move from consciousness to unconsciousness and back and forth; the sadhana helps push along the unconscious into the conscious."

Wade has also found that a harmonious balance between discipline and joy works its own way into sadhana during the practice itself. "B.K.S. Iyengar teaches that the pose begins when you want to get out of it, for me to stay conscious in sadhana, there's always an edge I have to play. That's why sadhana is so important because it is the anchor, the reconnection within, with all the distractions and forces pulling you outward."

In terms of assessing whether your sadhana practice is working for you Wade recommends looking at how your relationships are functioning. "Always make sure that your practice is helping you in cultivating relationships, in relationships with yourself, with other people and your community. I think that is an incredibly amazing gauge in knowing that your practice is working for you."

Yet ultimately Wade's advice for seeking out a sadhana to suit you is linked to joy. "Essentially, let your practice be something that you look forward to. Let your practice be something that grounds you. Let your practice be something that inspires you. Let it be something that you are excited to do."

That morning I would have run to my mat if I could have. When I got to it, my personal practice grounded me as I reflected on the synchronicity of the words shared with the lady who works in my local store. Yoga broke down barriers that led us straight to a deep topic of conversation; the sounds from her childhood still resonating within her so many years later, she shared that joy.

Chapter Three

Molly Lannon Kenny

A yoga teacher, yoga therapist, licensed speech-language pathologist, and musician, Molly Lannon Kenny is also an active member (Vice President) of the International Association of Yoga Therapists. Molly has developed a unique yoga based therapy method termed "Integrated Movement Therapy," that draws on her clinical and yoga background. Yoga classes, courses, workshops, retreats, and teacher trainings are all facilitated by Molly including the weekend-long workshop titled "Yoga and Social Change: The Power of Partnership." This three-day program educates participants about the unique and effective connection people within the yoga world can make with non-profit organizations to provide yoga to marginalized populations, and the link between yoga and social change and activism.

Molly is also the founder and executive director of The Samarya Center, a Seattle-based yoga studio that is "dedicated to healing our communities through yoga" by providing affordable yoga classes, specialized yoga training and community outreach yoga programs. Personally I'm not sure The Samarya Center could be situated in a better location. When I met with Molly, I traveled by train to downtown Seattle and then walked up a very steep hill to the center. The weather was mild enough to draw people out into the small parks, front yards, and neighborhoods I passed by, not in a crowded-city kind of way but in a thriving-community kind of way. As I walked, I passed many other people who seemed to be out in their community simply for the experience of *being* in it. Having reached the summit of my journey earlier than expected, I stopped for coffee at a café literally steps away from The Samarya Center. It was cozy, funky, and welcoming in a very laid-back neighborhood-like way. Either The Samarya Center buoys the energy of its surrounding city blocks with a light energy of joy, or the neighborhood attracted that kind of center. Maybe it just so happens that there are ley lines running under The Samarya Center's foundations emitting positive vibrations in the space above, or, perhaps, like attracts like, and it simply worked out well for everyone.

As well as keeping a busy yoga-related schedule, Molly has also played in rock bands all of her adult life, and she has been known to tell her students, "Yoga is punk rock," in the sense that what partly drew Molly to yoga and what she observes also attracts a lot of other people to it is that "it's a do-it-yourself experience; no one's telling you what you have to do and how you have to do it."

However, that sense of self-awareness and multidimensional autonomy is something that yoga and the development of a personal practice have brought to Molly's life. "I was one of those kids who was really flexible and physical. The grown-ups around me were always saying, 'You should do yoga,' but yoga didn't really mean anything to me. It was just a weird thing that some weird people did somewhere. Many years later I walked into a gym and saw a yoga class, and it sparked something. I decided, 'Oh, I'll try that.' It was an Ashtanga class, and I thought, 'Wow, I'm good at this. I seem like I can do this.' So actually, for quite a long time, I thought that Ashtanga yoga *was* yoga."

Molly became dedicated to the Ashtanga style of practicing, although a period of time passed before she came to understand the idea of yoga being linked to any kind of prevalent spiritual discipline. Molly was familiar with the overriding instruction of Pattabhi Jois, the Ashtanga teacher to, "Do your practice and all is coming," the advice continuing to fuel her dedication to the practice. However, as Molly explains, "I practiced but without having any larger context. Within that Ashtanga practice it can be very competitive and ego based, and so, to me, you practiced as much as you could because that's what you did to keep up with the Ashtangis."

However, Molly acknowledges that the benefits of her practice infused more than the purely physical aspects of her being. Linking the evolution of her practice to the development of The Samarya Center that she came to create, Molly explains that there's an interesting relationship between the two. "Even though I was only doing Ashtanga, and I was drawn to it because it felt like the first physical activity I'd ever done in my life that I was good at, when I was still working in a clinic, I would think, 'There's something about what I'm getting out of my yoga practice that would benefit the people in this clinic.' When I finally made the choice to quit my job in the clinic and try to somehow infuse my clinical practice with yoga, and I can say it now with enough distance, I would bring severely autistic kids or adult stroke survivors or head injury survivors, and I would try to teach them the Ashtanga series because that's what I knew. So I knew that there was something about yoga that could benefit other people, but the only tool I had was Ashtanga. So there was a slight, brief period of time at the very beginning when that was what I was trying to put together, so to me, that really tells me that even though I was doing this really competitive practice where nobody was talking about spirituality, that I was understanding something at some other level and even though I didn't know how to translate it, I had some kind of understanding."

Molly was attending a yoga therapy training course when she first became aware of the idea of a dedicated personal practice. After spending nearly four years dedicated to an Ashtanga practice, Molly became curious about the yoga experiences and practices of others. "I remember specifically asking people, 'But if you don't do Ashtanga, what do you do? You lay out your mat, and how do you know what you're supposed to do?' It didn't even occur to me that one would develop a practice that came from any kind of internal point of view. By the time I knew the word sadhana, I knew it because I had done a lot of my own studying and had become more and more interested in this bigger thing called yoga."

When Molly opened The Samarya Center many aspects of her life changed, including the way she practiced. She no longer felt welcome in her practice community and her practice of yoga in community changed to one of practice by herself. "Sadly when I opened this organization, I wasn't welcomed into my community anymore, and so I was left thinking, 'I don't know what I'm supposed to do now.' It was actually, as many things are in retrospect, hugely liberating because I would practice on my own. I would still be doing the primary and second series, and one of the most beautiful things that came out of that is that so many of the poses I had been fearful of, especially in the second series, suddenly I wasn't afraid of. I could actually do them with grace and ease, and they didn't seem as difficult as they had when I felt pressure to perform. I share responsibility with my teachers at the time, but I was certainly invested in the whole competitive thing. If you were on the mat next to me and you were 'better' than me, then a lot of my internal thought was, 'Okay, now I have to get at least as good as her if not better than her.' Of course, that's coming from a place that is not inviting ease in the body, so there was a lot of tension in the practice. Once I moved to a personal practice, I found much more ease, and then as I began to find that ease in the poses that I knew and the sequence that I knew, I naturally and organically started to deviate from the practice and do what I wanted to."

Molly's sadhana naturally and organically started to turn into a new style of yoga practice—*her* style of practice—and just as it *came* from her, it also *became* part of her and her daily expression of being. Thus Molly's personal practice became essential. "It's important for me because it's my life's work and it's my dharma. It very much defines who I am and what I do, not just professionally but in terms of my own spiritual development. I know, for example, when I don't sit in the morning, that my husband will sometimes say things like, 'Did you not have a chance to sit today?' So for my own mental health, it's important. Then to have the awakenings that I wish to continue to have throughout my lifetime, I've seen that a dedication to a practice is what would bring those things to me; so much happens, especially during meditation.

"I also think that especially with asana, with meditation too, but especially with asana, the best possible way for us to understand what might be going on in people's bodies, even down to something like nuts and bolts and how we move through transitions or how we talk about energy, so much of that has to come from our own felt sense. If we're not doing it, I don't know how any teacher can really authentically be teaching and specifically keeping their teaching fresh and new and something that is inspiring to their students."

This belief is held by Molly both as a guideline for her own teaching and for others. "I think all people who are teaching yoga also have to have a personal practice to keep their own selves on center and on track and to really continue to touch that spark that's motivating them to teach. One of the things I say to my teachers during teacher training is that I don't really care about teaching them to be yoga teachers. What I would like to teach them is how to be yogis, and if that natural flow is so powerful and so beautiful to them that they feel compelled to teach, then that's how that should happen."

Molly has noticed instances of this not being the case, and she finds that this results in the outflowing of the teacher and the information and experience shared in class not being the same. "I think that people doing their own practice is part of what keeps them very connected to that deeper source of inspiration that wants to share what's so beautiful and transformative for them."

On the front window of The Samarya Center is a picture of Molly in a rather impressive and complicated-looking arm balance pose. It comes across, though, as light and fun, not a symbol of what is expected of you if you come through the front door, but rather more a symbol of you being in good hands if you do choose to come to a class. This idea of balance, albeit figuratively, pervades Molly's perspective on how yoga classes can affect an individual's personal practice. "I've met lots of people now who learned yoga from a book or learned it from a video, and I'm always totally impressed with that because with my personal constitution, I don't think I could have done that. I think for many people, going to yoga classes is the only or the primary entrée they have into what might even become a personal practice."

Molly also observes that by trying to fit slots of sadhana time into our already hectic schedules in our busy lives in North America, we run the risk of that time getting eaten up by work, driving kids around, chores, and so on. Molly has found the structure of allotted class time can help to alleviate that issue, but she believes it's also important to maintain balance, be that literally or figuratively. As Molly explains, "The other side of the coin is that classes can be a hindrance because we start to rely on that yoga class as if that's the end, like that's where I want to get to, and as long as I can get to that yoga class, I've done my yoga. Maybe not enough teachers do talk about where else yoga happens and how else it happens. A lot of people don't know who is a good yoga teacher and who is not a good yoga teacher. If you don't have any basis for comparison, maybe the class is just 'okay.' "

To help you find balance in your own practice, Molly advises "going to different studios and different teachers and thinking about what would it be like if you rolled your mat out at your house and what might happen there."

Samarya is a Sanskrit word meaning "community." In yoga, when we come together in class in "communion," we can work to unify our efforts to connect both with a universal energy and with our fellow practitioners and to the universal energy within that we all share. For Molly, someone whose focus and life is very much rooted within community, taking time to practice alone is crucial. "I almost always practice alone. I grew up 'yogic-ally' practicing in community because I did that Mysore thing for quite a while, so that feeling of being in community and practicing together can be powerful." Occasionally, Molly schedules practice with her fellow teachers at The Samarya Center, and although she finds it fun and recognizes that there's a value to it ultimately, she acknowledges, "It's not what it feels like when I do my own practice."

Setting aside time for personal practice has helped sustain Molly as she cultivated and nurtured the community of The Samarya Center. "My practice has given me everything. It's given me levity, it's given me respite, it's given me joy, clarity, it's given me a healthy physical body. I have an awesome job, but there's a lot to keep in mind, and there's a lot to feel responsible for. My practice has given me a sense of everything slowing down and stopping in the best possible way, like a break and recalibration. It never takes away from my life; if anything, it's the other way around.

"I am really fortunate that I get to spend about three months out of every year at a house I have in Mexico with a yoga studio in the backyard. During that time I can wake up whenever I wake up and then go directly out to my studio and practice for however long I want. At some point in my life, I'd like to have that all year-round. I'd like to be able to give it even more time. Then there might be times where I go out to my studio and after forty-five minutes say, 'Okay, I'm done,' and it wouldn't be because I didn't have time; it would be because it felt done, it felt complete."

As the executive director and spiritual leader of The Samarya Center, Molly is mindful of not placing expectations of sadhana on her staff. "In many ways I deemphasize personal practice only because I feel like, in the world in general, there are so many different pressures, so many different ways for us to feel bad about ourselves, so many things that we're not doing that we should be doing. We should be eating this kind of food, we should be exercising this much, and we should be this productive and all of these things. Add the yoga community on, and now there are all these other sorts of expectations about what you should be doing, who drinks dairy and who doesn't, who's a vegetarian and who's not, how much you practice, and who meditates. For many people it's too much, and it becomes something that, rather than actually serving them, becomes just another thing that they feel that they can't meet."

That being said, Molly acknowledges that there is an aspect of discipline, even to a naturally evolving practice. At this point in Molly's life, the biggest challenge to her daily practice is traveling or a lack of structure in a busy day that leads to her being unable to schedule a reliable practice time. Keeping a specific routine time set aside for practice is a strategy Molly recommends for yoga practitioners who might sometimes struggle to find time for attending to their sadhana. "Anything that you want to do, structure is exactly what's going to bring you freedom. There are different constitutions, but for most of us, if our tendency seems to be flighty, for example, if I just say, 'Well I'll fit in my practice whenever I fit it in,' then most likely I'm not going to fit it in. If I don't sit in the morning and I think to myself, 'Well I'll just sit later on,' nine times out of ten it just never happens, and then I remind myself, 'That's right, that is nonnegotiable. You must sit in the morning.' That being said, I think we also have to get to a point where when you don't have the right room, you don't have the right music, you don't have your mat, it doesn't matter, you just figure out how you're going to do it."

Community is brought about by the balance of many contributing factors that create a gathered energy, a place, a feeling, a connection. Similarly, there are many aspects that can affect our linking with a sense of 'communing' within. As Molly explains, "I think we need to have that structure to create the discipline, and at the same time, we can't use that as sort of a crutch to say, 'Well, you know, since I don't have my special yoga room and my special yoga music, I guess I can't do it.' The only way that I practice shouldn't be because I have all my special accoutrements with me."

Self-awareness is essential in determining whether a practice is right for you or whether it should change or whether you need to simply apply more discipline. Molly describes the key signs that you're on the right sadhana path in the following way: "You look forward to it and you're excited and you're happy when you put your mat out. It feels like a natural flow, you don't have to think too much about it, you're just following your intuition. It doesn't leave you feeling exhausted or lethargic, nor does it leave you feeling overly amped up. There should be this beautiful state of clarity and balance that you experience and maybe when you miss your practice, you have a sense of, 'Oh, I missed my practice, I can feel that I missed it.' "

Molly makes a point of clarifying, though, that this doesn't mean you have free license to flagellate yourself for lack of foresight, scheduling, or effort. In the past Molly has experienced body-image issues and there were times when skipping a yoga practice might have been self-interpreted as skipping her workout. That perspective has long ago changed for her and evoked a more compassionate awareness of herself and of similar issues in others. "There should be a quality of 'I feel really good when I do that and I notice when I don't do it that I don't feel as good.' "

While Molly's yoga practice has gone through periods of self-guided transformation over the years, as much as there was a deep connection with self in order to bring about and generate this change, Molly also acknowledges the influence that many great teachers have had on her yoga journey. "Yoga is a really direct experience, and that's like the way punk rock is also really direct. Yet really, even to be punk rock, you can't say, 'I'm so punk rock that I'm not going to even put out any of my music ever, and I'm still going to become a famous rock musician,' or 'I'm so punk rock that I'm never going to play in a club.' In the same way with yoga, there's definitely a certain value in each one of us having our own experience, relying on our own intelligence and internal wisdom and becoming very comfortable with that and very trusting of that. Then I think that there's a certain point where I need someone to reflect back to me and to give me feedback about my growth or to show me a new way of looking at things or to challenge me.

"I think we can develop a beautiful soft practice, beautiful sadhana, completely on our own *and* with the benefit of a living teacher. I'm very discriminating about who that could be. That sense of humility and curiosity that comes with a teacher and getting that kind of feedback is really what will maximize our spiritual growth and our development. Yoga is do-it-yourself, it is punk rock in that way, but there are long time-tested things that work. We can do it ourselves, but we can also benefit from the wisdom of what's already been tested and what's already been shown to work, just in the same exact way that that's how I'm going to get my punk rock band to be 'The Sex Pistols.' "

Just as there are many kinds of music, not just punk rock music, there are also different styles of yoga classes and studios and teachers to choose from. Sometimes it can even seem a little overwhelming knowing where to start. Molly's advice is this: "Don't give up on yoga because the teacher wasn't good and don't stay at the first place that you find unless right away you're completely lit up. Allow yourself to look around and find a person who, when you're in that person's presence, you feel good; not just your physical body feels good but *you* feel good. Being in that person's presence feels uplifting to you. Conversely, if you're feeling in a yoga class that you are not valued or you're being pressured or you're being talked down to or there are hierarchies, trust your inner wisdom, you don't have to stay."

However, Molly advises that persevering with your personal yoga practice is worth the effort. "Stick with it, and the reward will be so much greater than you ever could have imagined. Really honor your own developmental process—honor your body and your heart on a day-to-day basis. The days when you feel really strong, do a strong practice. The days when you don't, take it easy. The days when your heart feels fragile, be sweet. See yourself as a human being doing a practice. Continue to seek a practice that feels like it's serving you and not that you're serving a practice."

There's a strength that comes from this inner awareness and a profound benefit from maintaining your well-being. Not to be shallow, but on a purely physical level there are many beautiful yogis and yoginis whom I meet who look far younger than someone in our culture typically might for their years, but, more important, they glow with health on many levels. I often wonder, on a purely physical level, why my grandmother looked infinitely older than my mother does at the same age. Some theorists put this down to a better diet, better lotions, and basically a better sense and ability of looking after ourselves now. My point is, with my generation—and the generation below me now as my children approach the teen years—what kind of long-range benefit will the profound influence and ever-growing practice of yoga have on our culture? Will even better health be bestowed on us in whatever way that might manifest or be expressed?

Molly is ten years older than myself, and she certainly doesn't look a day older than me (in truth, probably even younger), and she is far stronger physically (I have my own positive attributes too!) Molly acknowledges and appreciates the benefits that her practice is bringing her on a physical level as time passes. "The thing that hasn't changed and that's just a personal delight for me, or a blessing, is the feeling of physical competency and trust and gratitude for my physical body. My body is changing on the outside, and at the same time, there's a part that doesn't feel like it's changing on the inside.

"I have had very few injuries, very few limitations in that way. I remember practicing with a friend who was probably at least ten years younger than me and her asking, 'Do you think there's some age where you peak physically and then you have to scale everything back?' I just looked at her and laughed and said, 'Well I think there probably is, but you're certainly not at it. I'm not at it.' All the time I'm expecting that one of these days, I'm not going to be able to do a handstand or do whatever, but at the same time the thing that has changed is that things come more easily. I was over forty by the time I ever put my hands on the ground and decided I was going to press myself into a handstand. In some ways, I get stronger, but I think part of what that's coming from is I notice how much less I care. I have gratitude, and I'll do a hand balance and think, 'Look at me, I'm doing this hand balance.' When I was younger, I'd get mad if I tried to do a forearm balance and I couldn't stay up. There are some mornings when I do a forearm balance and I can't stay up, and I do it two or three times, and then I go, 'Alright, carry on to the next thing.' "

Ultimately it seems for Molly that sadhana comes down to living in truth on both a personal and a community level. "Yoga's not easy, and the spiritual path is not easy, and looking at your own 'stuff' is not easy. If your yoga practice is not bringing you more joy and more freedom and more sweetness, then it's not working. Yoga's a practice of freedom, and ultimately, what one should be experiencing, is a sense of greater ease and freedom, and if it's not moving in that direction, reassess."

The third Yoga Sutra explains that if our yoga is working for us, when we are united in heart, mind, body, and spirit, when a stillness comes to our being because of this, we live in truth, or rather more appropriately for Molly and The Samarya Center she has created, we truly live, and this community beacon of life, joy, and well-being is testament to the light inside.

Chapter Four

Gary Kraftsow

Gary Kraftsow began studying yoga with T.K.V. Desikachar in 1974 and went on to found the American Viniyoga Institute, of which he is both director and senior teacher. The American Viniyoga Institute offers private yoga therapy consultations, professional yoga teacher and yoga therapist trainings, retreats, workshops, and consultations for yoga-related research studies.

Receiving a Viniyoga Special Diploma from Viniyoga International in 1988, Gary also has a master's degree in psychology and religion, and is the author of *Yoga for Wellness* and *Yoga for Transformation*. Gary has also created the instructional DVDs *Viniyoga Therapy for the Low Back, Sacrum and Hips* and *Viniyoga Therapy for the Upper Back, Neck and Shoulders*, *Viniyoga Therapy for Anxiety*, and *Viniyoga Therapy for Depression* as well as the CDs *Chanting Live with Gary Kraftsow and Friends* and *Yoga Sutras of Patanjali—Chapter One* and *Two* (a commentary of the *Yoga Sutras*) and the *Yoga for Wellness* CD set.

Just before my scheduled interview with Gary, I was walking in my neighborhood and saw a sign advertising new classes being offered at a local yoga studio. It occurred to me that you often see yoga classes or workshops with a particular focus such as 'yoga for backs,' 'yoga for runners', 'core yoga,' 'prenatal yoga,' 'yoga for depression,' and so on, but I don't think I've ever seen a course offered anywhere along the lines of 'sadhana yoga,' or 'how to create a personal yoga practice.' Without a specific class focus, might it occur to yoga students that yoga tools can be used to address needs or wants specific to their body or disposition?

For some people, however, it seems that a conscious sense of self-awareness comes naturally. As a child, Gary sailed boats, and while some children might simply enjoy the experience, he came to understand life lessons through his sailing experiences, which continue to be linked to his sadhana. "Sailing was really my first sense of yoga because when you're racing on a boat, you're sitting. They're small boats, so you're holding the tiller, which is for steering, and the sheet, which controls the sail, and you have to look at the water and see where the wind is coming across the water. You're in the middle, and you're coordinating these discrete different things together, and through that ability to sense all these different elements, you're able to move things forward. Sailing was the first real yoga sadhana for me actually."

Not only did Gary garner a sense of how he could consciously apply different aspects of his abilities to control the progression of something when being mindful of the environment he was in, he also learned that practice itself was important. "When I was a kid, I went to camp in Maine, and I used to go sailing. I was on the racing team, and I remember that I was one of the best ones—the gold medal-type racer. When my friends asked me how I could do it so well, I said because my dad had a boat and I could sail all the time. So I had already known that if you do something consistently, your skill at it improves."

Gary's introduction to a more traditional practice of yoga came via an injury. "I was in high school, I think I was in ninth grade, and I was at a friend's house. I grew up on the East Coast of the United States, and my friend's mom was one of the very first yoga teachers in Philadelphia. I remember one time I was at his house, and his older brother showed us how to lift weights, and I pulled a muscle in my back. His mother put me in what I now know is vajrasana, or child's pose, and my back felt relief, but it came back again. His mother said, 'You know, you just have to do these kinds of movements every day for a few days,' and that was my first sort of insight about yoga."

There seems to have been an inherent manner of progression propelling Gary toward a more traditional yogic path as serendipitous, or perhaps karmic, opportunities began to come along at a more expedited rate as he matured and progressed into adulthood. "I did gymnastics in high school, and so I began to understand my body, and when I graduated high school, I went to Colgate University in upstate New York. I was in the religious studies department in the beginning, and I met a woman who was teaching yoga in the physical education department. She was actually one of the original Western students of Krishnamacharya. She had lived fifteen years in South India with her husband, who was an ethnomusicologist. He was out there studying carnatic music, and he was the chairman of the music department at Colgate University. I had a gym requirement, so I took the yoga classes, and there was an immediate recognition for me about practice. From the beginning in the Viniyoga that I was trained in, before I met Desikachar and Krishnamacharya, I was taught by her that you have to do this practice regularly or constantly. I had already done gymnastics and sailing, and so I knew about practice. I knew about the importance of yoga because it helped my back when I pulled my muscles, so I just got into it really from then."

Gary's more formal studies at the university also led him to discover and form a connection with yoga albeit from a different angle. "I started studying religion, and I ended up in a class on Hinduism and encountered the *Yoga Sutras* of Patanjali. That's when everything changed, and that was in 1973. It was actually in a religious library that I found the *Yoga Sutras* text. I asked my professor about it, and started studying them. Six months later, the yoga teacher and her husband were leading a study group to South India for carnatic music, and I asked if I could go. I wasn't a music student, but the requirement was that I did some, so I did South Indian drums. I arranged course work at Madras University, and I studied a particular tradition of Shaiva Siddhanta, which is a form of Tantra. I met Krishnamacharya, and I began studying yoga with him and his son Desikachar; that's sort of how it began."

Although exposed to yoga prior to traveling to India, Gary considers his formal concept of a personal practice using traditional methods of yoga, such as asana, pranayama, meditation, and so on, began in 1974 after immersing himself in yoga teachings during his time studying in India. Coincidentally, given the amount of fortuitous yogic interceptions that seem to have guided Gary to that point, one of his yoga teachers referred to him as a "Yoga Bhrashta." When Gary asked what that term meant, his teacher replied, "Don't think you know what you know about yoga from what you learned from me." When Gary asked him to explain, his teacher told him that he had been a yogi in a past life. "I died before I completed the journey, so I had to come back."

Although Gary's time spent sailing provides an experiential analogy for sadhana, his almost forty years of yoga practice and study have led him to a deep appreciation of the many aspects and effects of sadhana. "For me the word sadhana is very much connected to Patanjali's framing of it in the context of his first comments about sadhana in the Sadhana Pada, the second chapter of the *Yoga Sutras*, in the context of kriya yoga. Kriya in this context means action, and the great insight in yoga is that intelligence can influence the direction of change. Things are always changing, and so the great insight of yoga is that we can't stop change in the material world, but we can influence the direction of change through intelligent application of the right method. So for me, sadhana is that consistent intelligent application of the right methods to influence the direction of change in our lives. That direction of change is toward eliminating symptoms and causes of suffering and actualizing our higher potentials, leading toward, ultimately, finding happiness in the present moment and meaning and purpose in life in the face of the inevitable reality of change and impermanence and death.

"As a kid, my first insight of yoga was the idea that intelligence can influence change, as a gold medalist sailor seeing the reality that by paying attention I could win races. Then when I encountered yoga just a few years later, I realized that it's the actual science of how intelligence can influence change. You bring certain qualities to your present moment in your action and through that you can make your action be a ground for real transformation rather than just the typical action which follows pre-established patterns, which in yoga we call conditioning, or samskara. Kriya yoga is how action can actually create new and more functional patterns rather than just reinforcing existing dysfunctional patterns."

Yet sadhana for Gary is more than simply the application of the typical and traditional practice methods of yoga. "A lot of yoga in the West is focused not on yoga so much but on tools of practice. The root of the word 'yoga' is 'yug.' The actual cognate word that we use in common English parlance is 'to join.' The English word 'join' is actually the same root as the word 'yoga,' so, etymologically, 'joining' means 'to connect.' The other English word that we don't use in common parlance is 'yoke,' which is a particular tool that a farmer would use to attach the ox to the cart. The cart is the symbol of materiality, so you put your crop on the cart. The ox is the symbol of shakti, and you're connecting shakti to materiality. Then the intelligence is driving shakti, the product, to the market. So that's a beautiful image of intelligence harnessing and directing energy and then affecting change in the materiality.

"Yoga is fundamentally about that relationship between the consciousness and materiality and the idea of harnessing energy to change materiality. That happens when you're walking, when you're running, when you're washing the dishes, when you're sailing, or when you're doing sadhana in the formal sense; asana or pranayama, or chanting or meditation. I think that a lot of people have reduced yoga to some form of exercise and don't really understand that yoga is about the relationship to action, about consciousness relating to matter in this dance of life. The word 'Viniyoga' itself means 'intelligent application'; appropriate intelligent application to fit or suit the context in which it is being applied. Viniyoga, not uniquely, is among the few traditions that really are rooted in the deep understanding of yoga and its depth and breadth and draws on different tools but isn't focused on any tool. A lot of yoga is just focused on a tool."

If you're relying on a very subjective application of yoga tools, what might be the signs that you're cultivating an intelligent and appropriate sadhana? Gary believes that it will be reflected back to you on every level. "The first thing is that you should have less pain, not more pain, in your physical body. You should have more energy, not less energy. You should sleep deeper or feel more refreshed from sleep. Your digestion and elimination should be functioning well. Your cardiovascular rhythms should be more balanced. Your autonomic nervous system will be more in sympathetic/para-sympathetic balance. More importantly is that you should be happier. You should be less materially attached. You should be less judgmental, be more tolerant of others, and have a deeper sense of presence in your day-to-day life. When you're doing the right practice, then you become a more balanced human being and a more tolerant human being. If someone has a deeper understanding of yoga, all yoga can do is support all relationships. If you're not feeling happy or at least more content and more tolerant of others and less judgmental and freer internally and more at peace, then something is wrong with your practice."

However, that doesn't mean that the goal of your personal practice has to be the fulfillment of all the previously listed qualities. As Gary explains, "If you have back pain and you do a regular practice, you don't have to have back pain anymore, and that's fine, you don't have to be looking for enlightenment. Sadhana can be used for worldly aims or spiritual aims; it's all sadhana, and it's all valid. It has to do with an individual's dharma or svadharma. I think it's totally fine to use your sadhana to master asana so you can get a job in Cirque du Soleil or be in a picture in the *Yoga Journal*, that's a valid choice. You can use it for improving your back condition or sleeping better or dealing with anxiety or improving your memory or increasing your concentration or learning a different language. Yoga can help; you can apply yoga to help you achieve worldly ends, and it's fine.

"Sometimes I will use practice to help me understand something that one of my students is going through, or I will use practice to prepare myself before I go and do a keynote talk at the *Yoga Journal* conference in front of a thousand people. More recently, I had to do a talk in front of forty of the top executives in Fortune100 companies. I had to do something to prepare my mind and my nervous system to do that, so I used the practice to help me step into the world, but my deepest personal practice has to do with the inner journey of self-realization, and that's more like what you might call stepping out of the world."

In Gary's experience, having a goal or personal motivator can bring an ease of willingness to your practice of sadhana that might not always be effortlessly realized. "The obstacle to connection is distractions and patterns and desires and attachments. There is a deep paradox in yoga practice in terms of the yoga metaphysics because the metaphysics states that who we truly are is the unchanging source of pure awareness, and so we don't have to do anything to be that because we are already that. That has led to some confusion in that somehow sadhana is not important, but in fact it's more like a metaphysical model. Although it's true from the yoga perspective that we are Atman, unchanging source of pure awareness, we're identified with materiality, with the world, with our self-image and all of the things in the world that we're attached to and all our conditioned patterns.

"Sadhana is hard work; it's definitely hard work to maintain a personal practice because the television show we love is on or because you smell your neighbor cooking food or you want to play on your computer or do your work. You have to sacrifice your attachments in order to consistently maintain a personal practice. Although practice can be fun and can create a sense of deep well-being and pleasure or effectively help you get out of pain. People who have a lot of physical or psycho-emotional pain often are more naturally drawn to practice because they have a motivation. Although there is another group of people who just have a natural faith and desire to do this work. So there are those two categories, but it's not easy."

Gary's own application of yoga has resulted in the actuality of what his sadhana might look like to others changing greatly over the years. The *Yoga International* article "Radical Healing: Yoga With Gary Kraftsow" outlines Gary's experience of being diagnosed with a brain tumor, the subsequent surgery, his healing that followed, and how his application of yoga helped support him through those experiences. Having now experienced three brain surgeries, at times Gary's sadhana has been realized purely as a very conscious awareness of being. As he explains, "Before I went into surgery, I was doing whatever I could to keep my mind balanced and clear. I had a week when I realized that I would have to have major brain surgery before the surgery, so I was able to do a little bit of movement, but mostly it was pranayama and a lot of chanting and some meditation. After brain surgery, I couldn't move. I couldn't even do deep breathing, and I certainly couldn't chant because of the nature of my condition, but I could do a lot of meditation. Really it's the yoga that was important. It wasn't the specific tools; it was whatever I could do. So, in a case like that, I was doing more sadhana I think in the first month after my brain surgery than I've ever done. It was pretty much 24/7. I was constantly in that state of deep present awareness and meditation. There are some times in life where you're naturally drawn to sadhana, but when things are going well in ordinary daily life, sadhana is hard to get to because you have to really be committed to it, and it's a lot of work."

Despite this empathy for the challenges of upholding a commitment to a daily practice of yoga, however that might look, and an appreciation of how sadhana might evolve and mature, there are fundamental components of Gary's own sadhana that haven't changed during nearly forty years of practice. "Your sadhana isn't one fixed thing. There are core elements that persist throughout, but the sadhana constantly changes with time and circumstance and space availability. For me, the core thing that hasn't changed is self-reflection, the emphasis of increasing self-awareness in being present in the moment. The relationship between the flow of breath and the movement of the spine is the key element in all of my asana practice, attuning to my spine through the breath and using the breath to mobilize my spine. The ongoing study and chanting of yogic texts, principally the *Yoga Sutras* but also certain core Upanishadic texts, have been with me since really early on. I was a religious studies student, and I came to yoga from the perspective of a student of religion. Although I had done gymnastics, I didn't come to yoga through asana. I came to yoga through the study of Vedic culture and Vedic texts, and so that's been consistent. Mantra became important to me after I was really a little bit more mature. I was initiated into mantra in the early 1980s, so more than twenty-five years ago."

For as much as Gary had an instinctive connection with and reverence for yoga, he still benefited from opportune and relevant engagement with teachers and teachings that have helped shape his practice of yoga. While he believes that navigating and nurturing a wholly apt personal practice without guidance is possible, he also believes it is rare. "I think it's not impossible; it's just not common. The traditional view is that yoga is an initiatory process and the initiation is what empowers you to utilize the practices at a more deeply effective level. A traditional concept is that some form of initiation or receiving, what they call transmission, through a lineage that's alive, that's activated, is an essential part. I think it's possible that individuals can be self-directed and self-guided, but I think it's very uncommon. Reflect deeply about why you're practicing and what your motivation is to practice and then seek out teachers who seem to have not formulaic answers to your questions but who you feel are attuned to you and help you understand how the practices can support you where you are. They're not trying to shape you by making you do practices in a certain way but they're helping shape the practices so that they have more relevance to who you are and where you're going."

Gary has not personally experienced criticism for his dedication to a yoga practice. However, he appreciates that a commitment to a lifestyle path isn't always easy, and as aspects of our being or environment change, with or without conscious control, the reality of that change isn't always easy to live through and learn from. "The classic criticism of people who practice yoga sadhana is that they are self-obsessed or self-absorbed, and that's a misunderstanding. Although many people who do yoga are self-obsessed and self-absorbed and they get into the 'holier-than-thou, I'm a vegan, and therefore you should be a vegan' – they're yoga fundamentalists, and yoga fundamentalism to me is not any different than Islamist fundamentalism or Christian fundamentalism, and true yoga is not fundamentalism. It actually frees you from dogma and belief. True yoga enables you to actually be less self-obsessed and more present for others. My sadhana has worked in that direction. When I came back from India in 1975, and as I matured in yoga, certain people who were my friends I wasn't interested in anymore, but then I met other people who were interested in the things that I was interested in."

Looking back, though Gary's sadhana seems to have evolved naturally, if he could go back in time, he would ask himself to be a little more tolerant of others on their own journey. "Don't be attached to your ideas, and when people have different ideas, don't judge them; try to be present for them. When I was young, I alienated a lot of people by just speaking the truth. There were some growing pains for me obviously at having spent six months in India at nineteen with Krishnamacharya and Desikachar and then landing in the very beginning of the Ashtanga movement. I lived in Maui for thirty years, and Ashtanga really evolved in Maui after 1976, maybe 1978, after I'd come back from a couple of years in India. It took me a while to figure out how to handle what I understood in the context of that community and how to balance my own emotions in relation to recognizing that they hadn't been trained in the things I'd been trained in. I just knew too much at too young an age to have a healthy emotional relationship to it, and it took me a few years to go through that, to learn."

In the future, Gary foresees that he will continue to adapt his practice to suit his needs on many levels. "If I hadn't had the brain surgeries, I would expect that the natural progression for me would have been as I got older that I did slightly less intense asana and much more pranayama, with a growing focus on mantra and meditation. I was forty-nine when I had my diagnosis, and for two years they didn't want me to lift anything greater than ten pounds. Then I had another surgery in 2009, so there was a gap where I was just able to start doing practice again, stronger physical practice, and then I was told that I had to stop again. But I think I'm going to have to pick up my asana now because I'm getting past the third surgery, and I think it's better for my body to get more physically active again."

For someone whose life has incorporated actual encounters with mortality, Gary perceives a key role of the larger objective of sadhana as preparing us for the next realm of our existence. If we think about how we are shaping our sadhana in respect to the inevitability of that happening, especially as we get older, it may lend a greater purpose to our practice. As Gary explains, "There is this bigger question about meaning and purpose of life in the face of the reality of impermanence and death. The purpose of our sadhana is really for the moment of our death because the tradition says that where your consciousness is at the moment of death will influence what happens to you after you die. Of course the tradition says when you die, it isn't over, and what happens is very much connected to where your consciousness is in those last moments, in its last days or weeks or months. There's this very traditional perspective that the whole purpose of sadhana is to prepare us for the moment of death, and the condition of your hamstrings has got nothing to do with where your consciousness is going to be. The tradition says we should be thinking about our future lives and our sadhana is really to help us work through our karmic accumulations."

Chapter Five

Susi Hately

Initially attracted to yoga through the treatment of a sports injury, Susi Hately has been practicing yoga for over fifteen years and teaching for over ten. Susi has a BSc in kinesiology and a deep understanding of anatomy that, combined with her yoga experience and knowledge, has led her to develop a continuing education yoga teacher training program, a yoga therapy certification program, and a range of instructional yoga podcasts, books, and DVDs, including being a key contributor for the *3D Anatomy for Yoga: The Essential Guide*, a unique interactive reference guide to the anatomical aspects of asana. Through partnership with a research team at the University of Calgary, Susi worked to develop the *Yoga Thrive: Yoga for Cancer Survivors* program and instructional DVD set, and working with the Calgary Peter Lougheed Hospital, she has also developed a yoga program for individuals with idiopathic pulmonary fibrosis. Susi travels internationally, providing a comprehensive range of workshops, yoga, and yoga therapy trainings for both students and teachers and also delivers yoga training and educational programs online.

Susi is also one of those people you occasionally meet who has a truly fabulous laugh that really does light up a room: it's just a great laugh. She is passionate about what she does, and she exudes that in every facet of her being: her expression, her manner, and her honest communication of opinion and observation. I have to admit that I thought I was a type A personality until I met Susi. However, she has an ever-present underlying lightheartedness that bursts through the rhythm of her seemingly meticulous, conscientious, proficient, and poised sense of dharma, authenticated by a validity in her words and actions.

For Susi, her sadhana has become more than a personal practice; it has developed to become a way in which she lives her life. "I see sadhana as more than just personal practice. What I've come to know is that my yoga practice is never done, that I truly am never really going anywhere. The actual practice is about mastery, which is a combination of being the best me that I can be and growing into the best me that I can be, much like the quotation by James A. Michener: *The master in the art of living makes little distinction between his work and his play, his labor and his leisure, his mind and his body, his information and his recreation, his love and his religion. He hardly knows which is which. He simply pursues his vision of excellence at whatever he does, leaving others to decide whether he is working or playing. To him he's always doing both.*"

There was a natural, instinctive connection to yoga from the very first class that Susi attended, although at first she was a bit unsure of the experience. "I had one of those light bulb moments in the first class I went to, and I'll never forget it. My class was in a church, and whilst standing on my mat, I had no clue what I was getting into. I looked around at the other people wondering if they knew what they were getting into. As the class got going, I was told that Tadasana is the classic asana, the foundation of all asanas. All I could think was, 'What have I gotten myself into? I'm standing!' But something happened in that class, where I felt myself thinking, 'This is it . . . this is it.' "

This instinctive affinity for yoga led to Susi implementing a personal practice because of the benefits she experienced when she practiced as opposed to striving to fulfill an obligatory and disciplinary routine. "I've never seen it as having to have one from a necessity standpoint. It just has made life more fulfilling because all of my life is that. Have you ever had the experience of knowing that something was just right? It found me."

This organic connection that Susi trustingly nurtured through continued yoga practice started to bloom into other realms of her life. "About a year into practice, I started having moments of, 'Wow, I could actually do this for a living.' I had no idea how, I had no idea when or where, but there was such a fulfilling piece that I was experiencing, a piece I didn't get from any other work that I performed. So I just kept practicing, and all the other pieces fell into place. For example, when I moved to Calgary, I happened upon a 'Kinesiology of Yoga' workshop hosted by an Indian yogi. I thought, 'Wow, I love both those things.' Partway through the workshop, I decided that I was going to study with him in two years. Two years later I was in Pune studying with Dr. Karandikar, and when I got back, I started teaching full time."

Throughout the classes, training, workshops, and self-guided learning Susi has completed, she has meshed together the essence of their benefits and applied it in a way best suited to her own needs. Yet, while her personal practice may have evolved and matured with her over the years, there are also key core elements that have held their place in the foundation of her sadhana. "The only thing that has changed is a recognition to do the components of practice that I need in a certain moment. When I first started, my practice was very much about asana. Then I learned that asana practice was merely a way to get one prepared for meditation, which led me to become curious about, 'Well, what the heck am I getting prepared for? What's this meditation thing?' As my interest in meditation grew, my practice shifted from solely an asana practice to asana and meditation or a sitting practice. I love the combination of the two, and over the years this combination has ebbed and flowed. For example, last year I fell down the stairs, and I landed on my coccyx and was unable to move or sit. My asana and sitting practices shifted into nonasana/nonsitting practices. I became very introspective and very quiet. It was in that quiet that I healed."

One of the ways in which Susi's sadhana has somewhat transformed is her perception of its purpose. Susi's steadfast rhythm of achievements in her career are not only balanced out but also sustained by her softening of expectations of sadhana and a slowing down of her personal yoga practice. "There's a richness to the practice where I feel like I get to point at the moon, knowing that I'll never get to the moon but also knowing that it's not about getting to the moon. For people who think it is, they are missing out on the real juice of it. I understand their thinking since I used to have similar thoughts. The transition from those thoughts was definitely a point of maturity for me. There was a moment of time when I simply realized it really wasn't about getting anywhere, so why not move and live life with more ease, more grace, and less tension? As soon as I had that insight, something very interesting happened: I saw that the slower I approached life, the faster I actually achieved my goals—and here is the world-class piece—with a lot more grace, ease, and fun. In essence, the journey revealed itself, and the achievement of my goal—it was mere window dressing. I share this with my students very regularly since many of them are goal oriented and often fixated on production. I show them how to pull back and breathe and 'let the yoga do its work.' Every single time the world opens up, and all of a sudden their work just gets done or the next level gets reached or whatever it is that they're yearning for actually comes to them with a lot more ease. It is almost as if the moon is shining on them."

This "softening" of her sadhana practice provided a point of realization for Susi early on in her yoga training that resulted in her quickly becoming attuned to the needs of her physical body. "I came to yoga with pain, unable to do the activities I loved to do. After four months of yoga, I was able to run a ten-kilometer race pain free. More importantly, though, during that race something happened; I don't know what it was, but I still remember thinking, 'Wow, I'm different.' In fact, that whole four-month period after that first yoga class was different. I remember going out for a run and literally running around the block. I still remember coming around the fourth side of the block thinking, 'This is really weird. Why am I only going for a run around the block?' But I knew that's all I could do. I was being more thoughtful with how I was approaching exercise.

"About four weeks into my yoga classes, I remember the yoga teacher saying to me, 'You have hard feet, and you need to soften your feet.' I smirked and nodded, but five years later, I became aware of my very hard feet, and with that awareness I was able to soften them. The feeling was immediate, and I got a whole lot lighter in my running and in my life. It's that which has kept me on path; I kept seeing the result of getting further, of getting faster, of experiencing less strain and more freedom. It happened every time I applied asana and every time I chose ease over tension. With those results, I bought in hook, line, and sinker, and it is as remarkable today as it was those many years ago, whether I see my own students integrating the concepts or the students of the teachers I have trained. It wasn't just me having these very cool, almost radical experiences. It was the concept of yoga that was at play."

Just as Susi considers the concept of sadhana to extend to more than simply the time spent on her yoga mat, similarly the personal benefits that Susi has experienced through yoga have not been gleaned exclusively through what is sometimes referred to as a "home practice." "I don't know if a home practice is the gold standard. I think the gold standard is doing the practice that serves you, whether it's a home practice, or a workshop once a month and a home practice or going every day to a studio. There are a lot of people who don't have a home practice, but they're living their yoga. I've experienced times of moving from a home practice to a studio practice; sometimes I find that I need to be in a group with a teacher teaching me."

Just as the benefits of yoga are not necessarily exclusively acquired during the time spent alone in practice, lessons we experience that help us to mature and learn as human beings are not limited to occurring on a yoga mat. However, the way that we comprehend those moments or experiences in life can determine whether it becomes a developmental aspect of our greater expression of sadhana, something Susi has firsthand experience of. "If we broaden the term sadhana to mean something beyond yoga, I think the guidance we are seeking or needing doesn't always have to come from a yoga teacher. I think it can come from any kind of mentor. I believe that yoga is a set of organic principles and there are people out there who aren't practicing yoga but live according to these organic principles. They have a lot to teach and can provide a fresh look at the practice, which can sometimes get caught up in doctrine. The key is that they need to be people who really do preach what they practice. Are they truly eating their own cooking? At its essence, I believe I can't teach anybody anything I'm not willing to do myself. When I meet someone who could be a mentor or who could be a teacher, I am looking for them to share that theme."

When looking for signs that your more traditional yoga practice, whether it is cultivated in class or at home, is the best application of yoga for you, Susi recommends taking a more practical and tangible reading of the results of your efforts. "There needs to be a result of having more internal calm versus chaos. We all know what that feels like; it's not something that you can fake. That's not to say that you will always be serene or you will always be calm and you won't have chaos; that's not the point. It's that when you are in those moments of chaos, you'll simply notice, and out of noticing you'll experience those moments with more ease or you'll be more conscious. As a result, you'll probably find a way out as opposed to getting totally stuck."

For Susi, this mindfulness of being can be applied to every level of practice, and in terms of asana, it denotes the difference between mindless movement into yoga postures and mindfully being in yoga asana. Susi is passionate about anatomy—about movement and our awareness of our functionality and ease in the when and how we move. Through her own practice and observations of how other people move and practice yoga and complete exercise, she defines the difference between yoga movement, yoga asana, and exercise in the following way: "Asana loosely translated is 'sitting comfortably and still,' whereas typically an exercise program is not. I know a lot of people who practice yoga and who apply yoga to their exercise program, for example, running. When they run, they are approaching each step as if they are 'sitting comfortably and still,' so in effect they are in asana practice while running. I know other people who run and are not in asana whilst running; instead, they are in tension and in strain. So, depending on who you are and how you live, there could be an absolute distinction between a true asana practice and exercise practice. Then it also could be that, for some people, they are in asana when they exercise. We could use the same train of thought with yoga classes at many studios, which are often exercise programs that are built up of yoga poses. As a result, there are a lot of people in those studios who are not in asana; instead, they are simply in yoga postures. In these instances, yoga has become an exercise regimen, a string of yoga postures which a body moves through. To me this is no different than running, it's no different than swimming, it's no different than hiking: they are all movements. The key is the 'how' of how we approach it that brings forth the asana.

"I will receive emails from yoga teachers saying, 'I have sacroiliac joint pain, and I don't understand why; I do yoga.' I will respond to them, once I know them well enough, with, 'The reason you have sacroiliac joint pain is because you do yoga.' As yoga practitioners who have been practicing for a long time, we've had the opportunity to have witnessed miracles; we've seen students transform in amazing ways. As a result, we can often develop an inappropriate admiration for yoga believing that yoga is this magical thing. We have to remember that when we're doing handstands, we are performing movement; planks are movement, downward dogs are movement. The questions we need to ask are, 'How are we doing downward dog? How are we doing handstands? How are we doing plank? Why do we get torn hamstrings? Why do people blow out their knees? Why do people harm their wrists?' It's the way, it's the how. Ultimately, I think that this is an Eastern style of movement and Eastern philosophy of movement, and we have a Western mind that is trying to do it 'right.' Our Western mind has been influenced by the Jane Fonda 'no pain, no gain.' We have to remember that just because someone's doing triangle pose doesn't mean they are doing yoga. That's why there is the word 'asana,' 'asana' as opposed to 'yoga posture,' because it's that component; the necessity of 'sitting comfortably and still' as opposed to with tension that is so vital to the practice of yoga."

This idea of striving to seek out ease in action, both physically and philosophically, is exemplified in the compassionate kindness and honesty that pervades Susi's pragmatic point of view in terms of sadhana advice. "I think people can get caught up in the term 'practice makes perfect' or 'perfect practice makes perfect,' and really there's not much truth in those phrases. What is true is that sort of phraseology pushes people away from the mat. The key is to remember that the first step is to get on to the mat—just get on it. People come to see me and say, 'I need an hour program, and I need to do it five days a week because I want to have a daily practice.' I look at them and ask, 'Are you sure? How much time do you really have?' and then as we talk what will emerge is they have twenty minutes, three days a week. They'll ask, almost desperately, 'Is that enough?' and I'll say, 'Yes. Why not work with what you've got in your life, rather than trying to shoehorn something into your life?' If you do, your life will open up. The key is about making an initial change, not dissimilar to any other kind of change, like losing weight. If we go too hard at it, it won't be something we can integrate."

Just as Susi advises that people integrate their yoga practice into their life in a realistic way so that the potential is there for it to develop naturally rather than in a forced manner, the benefits of her sadhana continue to bloom in both a naturally lucid and a harmonizing way. "I think my practice has helped me see with new eyes. I love the analogy of wearing sunglasses and noticing they are dusty and being able to wipe off the dust. My practice is often about wiping that dust off. For example, there are times when life calls and there are struggles or there are complaints. It's during those times that my practice becomes very rich. Whether it's on or off the mat, I have a lot of patience and containment to be able to sit in particular struggles or complaints because I ultimately know that that struggle or complaint exists for me to learn, so I sit in the tapas and watch what unfolds. Over the years, my practice has given me containment so not only does lead, the struggle, transform into gold, freedom and wisdom, but I am able to see with new eyes and a more refined sense of patience. I think sometimes people feel when they get into struggle that 'this is not the way life should be,' but that is exactly what life can be; the key is how we place meaning on it."

Lessons in life come in many different forms, but Susi believes that yoga can help us understand how the effects of our experiences can be felt in every facet of our being; that there are daily occurrences that illustrate our body/mind/emotion/breath/spirit/energy connection. Susi's awareness of and respect for that unification has helped guide her choices in a positive and at times healing way. "Right after I fell down the stairs and I slammed my coccyx, I was in so much pain. I remember trying to stand back up and thinking, 'Holy $%# this is sore. I am sore.' As the days and weeks progressed, I was exhausted. I couldn't practice, and I couldn't sit. However, I trusted the process enough to know that I wanted to get back to my practice and I wanted to be well. I didn't want to be one of those people who practice in pain because a) it is not what I teach my students and b) I knew from experience that approach wouldn't work. That was on a physical level, but there was also the mental/emotional realm. I remember this one moment where I was sitting all propped up doing some work and complaints were going through my head—complaints about life, complaints about my current situation—and I knew that I was just so right about those complaints, like I was *right*. Then I had a realization. When I was ruminating, I could feel my pelvic floor tightening up around my coccyx. I thought, 'Okay, so I think I'm right, yet there is an incongruity going on in my physical structure.' So, as I have these overwhelming 'I am right' thoughts, my body is saying, 'No you're not because if you were truly right, then I'd be open and free and I wouldn't be in pain or in strain.' So I became really quiet and asked, 'Okay, do I really need to be right about this? Can I let this go? What is more compelling for me right now: to be right about it or to be back to my yoga practice?' It was literally in that instant when I loosened. I can laugh and say that I really was right about those scenarios, but the attachment to being right and making another wrong or making the situation wrong was gone. What remained was an element of connection between a thought in my mind, an experience of that thought through my body, and then a realization: 'Wait a second, this is a more compelling option.' "

While sadhana may have cultivated a connection to a viewpoint that seems more rooted in a comprehensive observation of her own reality of truth, this clarity of being able to make choices anchored to authenticity or that promote her well-being on different levels isn't always the easiest compass to use to guide your way through life choices, yet it ultimately leads to moving through life with ease. "Sometimes getting real can be hard to face at first. I say that sarcastically because sometimes in getting real, there is an awareness of, 'Wow, I'm really attached to that,' and truly that realization, at times, sucks. My body is saying one thing, and my mind, my brain, is saying another thing. There's that moment of truth, a speechless moment of, 'Wow, alright, maybe I'm not so right,' and then literally the next moment is one of, 'Alright, since I am more compelled to do this than this, I can let this go. I don't need to have this attachment.' I ultimately find that when I get real about things, whether it's in my own body or whether it's with my assistant or with any of the mentors that I work with or anyone else in my life, there is a greater and better result. The key is to first notice and move through that first initial blast of 'realness,' and when you do, there is progress."

While sadhana, big picture, or in terms of time spent on her mat in a more traditional practice of yoga may have revealed many messages and signs to Susi, her years of practice have provided her with a resiliency, security, and clarity not only to be able to listen effectively but to also determine whether best to let go of attachment to an issue, to learn to simply sit with it, or to take action to resolve those concerns and, if so, how best to go about it. "I've had so much experience over the past number of years that I'm willing to feel fear and be with it because my body doesn't lie to me. If my guts are in a knot or if my tailbone is sore or my breath gets held, that's a sign for me. I don't necessarily know what it means, but it's a sign to let me know that something's up. Then I sit quietly and ask, 'Okay, why are you here? What is it that you want from me today? What do you need? What action do I need to take?' These are great guiding questions to help in developing and trusting the wisdom of my body. Sure I realize it may sound goofy to some people; there are so many advertisements that don't honor the body's intelligence. Instead, they are basically saying, 'You are in pain or you are sick, but if you take our medication, you can keep busting through life,' but if you really think about it, isn't our body, in these scenarios, actually communicating something to us? It is curious really. It is interesting that we haven't been taught how to pay attention to the sensations of our body, to pay attention and listen and not to grapple with what they are meant to mean, to not try to figure it out, but rather to simply sit and allow for the unfolding.

"When people learn this, they feel they have touched on a brilliant little secret. The intelligence of their body becomes their guide. It's just brilliant. Think of all those times where you haven't said something that you've really wanted to say and you maybe got a sore throat or a headache or a gut ache. For some people, it is their foot that gets sore, or they might get tight or constrained or bloated or whatever. The key is not so much *where* the tension is held but rather that there *is* tension. There's something in the tension, there's something that's getting your attention, and if you choose to, you can be guided by it."

Susi teaches that mindful personal practice, a tuning in to what your own body or greater world might be trying to tell you, is not unattainable and does not have to be perfected as a practice to be efficient. "It doesn't have to be perfect. You don't have to have all the props. You don't even need to have a yoga mat. You don't need to have a meditation cushion. You just need to do it. You don't need a lot of time. You just need to start. If someone does it authentically and true, then they'll experience the rich results from it."

Chapter Six

Doug Swenson

Doug Swenson has been studying yoga for over forty years. With mindfulness and experience he has selected and blended aspects of varying traditions of yoga to cultivate what he has named "Sadhana Yoga Chi." The author of *Yoga Helps*, *The Diet That Loves You Most*, *Power Yoga for Dummies,* and *Mastering the Secrets of Yoga Flow*, Doug has also created the *Deep Relaxation* CD. Taking a holistic approach to both his personal practice and his trainings, workshops, and retreats, Doug's connection to nature and its energy is reflected in his words, actions, and day-to-day being.

Doug spent his early childhood years in Texas, and it was Dr. Ernest Wood who helped to plant a sense of sadhana for him at a young age. "The first two years I did yoga, I didn't know I was doing yoga. My parents belonged to a church group called the Unitarian Fellowship, and it was kind of a loose-knit group of people with different ideas, different concepts. One of the members of the group was Dr. Ernest Wood, and he was a yoga master. When I was thirteen every two or three Sunday school weekends he would teach us some yoga, some posture, and some meditation, but when you're young, you do it but you don't realize you're doing it. I would do it, and I remember how it felt afterwards, especially after meditation. I remember the first time I did a headstand; it just felt so different afterwards.

"Two years after that, I was only fifteen, but my parents allowed me to go to California one summer with some older friends of mine and my sister's boyfriend because I wanted to go surfing. I was surfing in a place in southern California called Swami's, and when I came in from surfing there was a big beautiful building on the bluff there, and some people on the lawn were doing some of the things that Dr. Wood had taught me. I went over and asked them what that was, and they said, 'It's yoga.' All of a sudden a little light came on in my head and went, 'Well, I do yoga.' It was the Self-Realization Fellowship founded by Paramahansa Yogananda, in Encinitas, California."

Having connected with this more formalized practice of yoga, Doug was determined to let his interest in yoga practice evolve. Although Dr. Wood had passed away, Doug returned to the roots of his practice and sought out Dr. Wood's teachings through his books and began to develop a personal yoga practice. It deepened Doug's connection with nature, both the nature of himself and his environment. "I just practiced out of his books every day by myself. From then on, pretty much I did yoga consistently with very few breaks. It just came naturally to me. I always did other things, and I was just a little kid at the time, but my yoga became my surfing, my surfing became my yoga. I was living in Texas at the time, and Texas doesn't have very good waves, but, in spite of that, I went on to go to the World Surfing Championships. It was because of my yoga, not just the flexibility but the sense of being able to connect with the energy of the ocean, and to feel a sense of awareness when I'm out on the water."

Doug continued to blend his interests and practices that seemed unquestionably interconnected to him, despite sometimes being advised to the contrary. "I think yoga is more than just posture and reading something out of a book; it has to do with your daily intentions. I've had people tell me, 'You can't do other things; you've got to just do yoga. If you run or surf or something, that's not yoga,' but to me, it's all in how you approach something or your consciousness when you're doing it. I would cross-train with other concepts, like walking meditation, like hiking, or anything that involved interacting with nature."

Out of his continued yoga practice, inquiry and connection with other practices, teachings, and ways of connecting with the world around him, Doug came to develop an approach to yoga that he terms Sadhana Yoga Chi. "How that came about was I practiced a lot of different styles. I like to try different things, and I've never found one style that seemed like it had the whole package of exactly what I was looking for."

However Doug continued to explore what a personal yoga practice could look like. "When I first started practicing yoga, I just assumed everyone who did yoga was doing the same thing. Then when I finally found a yoga studio in Houston, Texas, where I was living, it was a little bit different to what Dr. Wood presented in his book. I thought, 'That's kind of nice,' but that didn't last too long, just a number of months. The first organized style I did was Sivananda yoga. The softer styles of yoga were my best, like Sivananda yoga and Integral yoga. I used to go to Kundalini yoga, but at that time, I didn't want to say, 'Okay, I'll just do Kundalini yoga and not do Sivananda yoga or not do Integral,' because I liked parts of each.

"Then I moved to California, and I started doing Iyengar yoga with Ramanand Patel and that's when I was exposed to Ashtanga yoga. I tried to commit myself to Ashtanga yoga for three or four years, but most of these styles tell you don't do anything else because it is a distraction. I just couldn't buy that. I was doing Ashtanga yoga, but every few days I would go off and do my own thing, which was actually a complement because it provided an easier access to a different sort of flow because of the unique way that I move between postures. To me it's like moving energy. It's not just how I get from A to B, it's conscious—you're moving energy. Most people think, 'Okay, I'm in this pose, I'm going to go to that pose,' and they don't think about what's happening in between. They just go to the next pose."

Doug believes that the focus of practice is to connect with a flow of energy, not to merely execute or express poses. "No matter what you do and who you are and what kind of car you drive, when you come into a yoga class, everybody tries to find that place where they're connected to some natural flow of energy. A lot of times we get distracted by, 'Look, Billy has his legs behind his head,' or, 'Sally can really sit in lotus good,' and the posture itself is just a catalyst to connect with something, to connect you with that natural form of energy. There are so many franchised systems of yoga, but a lot of times, it's like a fish in the ocean looking for water. A lot of times people are looking here, looking there, and it's all around them. A lot of people don't realize that."

Doug continued on his sadhana path, selecting and blending what he had absorbed from different practices to best serve his sadhana and teaching needs, which understandably led to change through his decades of constant yoga practice. "My approach to things has changed. I used to think the more, the better. Now it's more like quality instead of quantity. It used to be too that I felt like if I found a new yoga posture, I had to do that one too and I kept building, building, building, until my routine got too big. I felt like I was being disrespectful if I didn't do every pose, every day. Now, it's like all days are interlaced, so as long as I have something positive that I can gain out of my yoga practice, I don't have to necessarily do every pose all the time."

For Doug, his sadhana is inherent in the way he lives his life. "As I get older, I realize that everything is interconnected and interlaced and that yoga is an internal practice with external results, so what you do reflects throughout your life. If you get frustrated with the yoga practice one day, you're going to be frustrated in life, and sometimes you just have to be at peace with where you are. My yoga has become an art form, physically and mentally. I view it as being something more sacred in a part of the grander scheme of things where it used to be just something that I did for an hour or two a day, separate from everything else. It's all connected—you find the energy in the trees, in the grass, and in the wind, and you try to bring that back into your yoga practice."

Yet surely we all have days when our yoga practice just doesn't seem quite the same. While we place effort to connect with that flow of energy, it seems to elude us. Doug believes that there is still a benefit to those practices, even if it feels like you're not quite achieving the desired effect. "My brother and I used to call it 'being in the zone.' We would have days when we would do yoga, and we would go through all these poses, and they might be impressive to people, but we'd call it a no-yoga day if we didn't get in what we call 'the zone.' It wasn't a waste of time because everything is a learning experience. Other days, the practice might not be that impressive, but you're really mindful and you're connected, and it clears a lot. Whether you call it success or failure or whether you get connected or don't get connected, it's all part of growing."

That's not to say that Doug believes sadhana is limited to time spent on a yoga mat or in meditation or however your personal practice of yoga tools might look. Just as Doug teaches his students the importance of how you move in between poses is still a part of your yoga practice, similarly off the mat it can be in those in-between times where much of life happens. As he explains, "Your whole life is one big vinyasa, and then the events are the poses, like the time you got married or you climbed a mountain or you bought a new car, but something happens in between those times and if you have no conscious awareness of what's going on in between times, it's like you're wandering around lost. The journey is everything. Say you're climbing a mountain; if it was just being there, somebody could drop you off there in a helicopter, and you could go, 'Wow, this is cool,' but it was that effort and energy and experience to get you there. It's the same with the yoga postures if you were just in a pose and doing the pose; it's the progress that gets you there."

You know when you're walking on a beach or hiking in the mountains and you see a sheer rock face battered by waves or a waterfall or wind and you spot a beautiful flower or defiant tree extending out to life, and you think, "Wow, look at that—how did that manage to grow *there*?" Possibly there is something innate in that particular seed or sapling, or perhaps just a strange yet opportune instance of a fertile environment occurred or maybe a force greater than itself willed its existence, or a mixture of all these things, yet it seems misplaced—not quite embraced by its greater surroundings.

Similarly, in Doug's younger years, his environment didn't always provide the most supportive circumstances for developing a personal yoga practice. "I know that because of the geographical region my brother and I were raised in, we were going against the grain 99.9 percent of the time there. There were one in a thousand people who did yoga where we were raised."

Yet, despite his surroundings, Doug's sadhana thrived, but you can't help wonder why that was. What made Doug confident enough to carve out a different path for himself? Doug explains, "I know that Dr. Wood's influence helped. I think because I was raised in a really conservative area, where there was a dress code and the way you dressed and wore your hair had to conform with that, I started questioning all of these things. Even to this day, if something is written in a document, I still like to think, 'Well why is it that way?' It started when I was really little because yoga is supposed to be expansive and open your mind and broaden it and keep evolving. Yet sometimes, in the yoga community, people feel like, 'This is what I'm looking for, and I don't want to see or hear anything else.' I think because of where we were raised, it helped my brother and I to be a little bit more flexible mentally."

Although Doug had a companion on his yoga journey in his brother David and his parents supported his interest in yoga, Doug was still at times viewed as deviant for practicing yoga, resulting in him being not only harassed in public but also in being arrested. "I would do yoga outside a lot because it was a warm climate. I didn't have access to studios, so I'd just do yoga in the park in our neighborhood, and I did yoga there every day for quite some time. Then one day a couple of the neighbors were concerned, and so they called the police. The police came and asked me what was going on, and I said I was doing yoga. They got really upset and handcuffed me and took me to jail, and that was it. I think people thought it was against the grain of religion or something."

Doug encountered a similar experience when promoting a yoga book he had written. "I published a book in 1974 called *Yoga Helps*. The reason that evolved was that I was in an automobile accident, and I broke my leg. From that I had a small insurance settlement, so I used the money to publish *Yoga Helps* because yoga really helped me physically and mentally recuperate from the accident. My brother helped me do a demonstration out in front of a bookstore in a shopping mall with their blessings. We had a little stage built up, and one of us would do a yoga demonstration and the other would narrate, and I had my books for sale there. The security guards came and grabbed us. They wouldn't listen to what we were saying; they handcuffed us and took us out and we had to get the bookstore manager to escort us back in. We were there with the blessings of the bookstore, but people just see something that's different, and then they get nervous. So that's just sort of the environment we were raised in, but because of that I became very independent. There are a lot of people in yoga who are flexible but not that many who have flexible minds. I was raised in an environment where I had to be my own example of what was positive because most of the people around me were always trying to pull me in different directions."

Sadhana has played a key role in Doug's personal growth, providing him with a way of checking in with whom he really is when the outside world may not always have been reflecting that back to him or even being tolerant. "When I step on my mat, it's like when you get out of your car and you step your feet onto the city park. You know that everyone goes there to be relaxed and to feel at peace. It's similar to that when I step on my mat; that is the time to really focus and be more connected. I always tell my students to bring that with them when they step off the mat. It's a constant reminder. It's like when you're in a traffic jam and you're upset about the traffic. But then you see a beautiful sunset, and you go, 'Ah, that's kind of nice.' You might not have seen it otherwise because you were too busy going somewhere but then you were stuck and you were forced to look at it. On the mat, it is right there in front of you, and you go, 'Okay, I am standing on this mat because I'm trying to get my physical, mental, and spiritual union.' We're always trying to remind ourselves why we're here and what's important. That's why they call it yoga practice because if you could just do it once and it could all be fixed, you wouldn't need to do it the next day. Then they wouldn't call it yoga practice; they could call it yoga done."

In his writings, Doug encourages readers to be mindful of how they fuel their body and nourish their internal nature. Yet while Doug expresses his passion about this subject eloquently, he has a sense of humor about it. On his website, Doug advises, "When you get hungry and find yourself staring down the barrel of a sugar donut, armed with a full mug of hot coffee, preparing to declare war on your whole anatomy, be sure to remember your body is your temple and you should treat it with respect."

Doug does not perceive a compassion and connection to both internal and external nature as separate. "I think it's all interlaced. It's like your body is your temple, and if we just eat junk food all day long, it's disrespectful to it. The body is just a vehicle, and we are just wearing this coat for a while, but at the same time, if your body is your temple, why would you want to throw a bunch of trash and garbage in there? Energetically, everything is all interlaced. The tree has a consciousness, the ground has a consciousness, the Earth has a consciousness, and we have a consciousness. To think we are a separate entity is a little selfish or egotistical. To me, it's all interlaced. Your thoughts create seeds, and what you eat, drink, and think becomes you. If you eat bad food, have erratic stray thoughts, and drink something that's not functioning well in your body, then you never feel your full potential basically. What people eat, what they drink, where they go, and who they hang out with becomes their demeanor, and that becomes their thoughts, and the thoughts become the action.

"It's like going out into the woods and you see a deer eating grass and drinking river water and the sunlight's sparkling down and then you smell something behind you. You turn around, and there's another deer smoking a cigarette, drinking a coffee, and having a sugar Danish and you go, 'What are you doing? You should be out here.' That deer is sitting on the porch of his little house and says, 'No, I'm not. That's not natural. I can't be like that. That's extreme. That deer over there, drinking river water and eating grass, that's crazy.' It's like humans—we put ourselves in these little tin boxes and drive around, we sit in houses, and we read books but the real thing is out in nature."

However, you can have too much of a good thing. Just as nature is sensitive to stress and functions well when balanced, so Doug is mindful of maintaining balance within his yoga practice. "As far as the yoga asana, if you do too much, it has the reverse effect where you feel lethargic and negative. That's why nature to me is an uplifting thing. Sometimes I'll take off from the formal asana practice itself or from reading a book and go out. To me, hiking is yoga and surfing is yoga and biking is yoga. If I'm doing yoga outside, I am more consciously aware of things and can appreciate them a little bit more. I think people should take off for a bit and then come back to it. They'll find it more enjoyable and they'll get more out of it. That is what has kept me doing yoga so long. I've had friends where it was all or nothing, and then they just quit altogether."

This philosophical flexibility and willingness to transform seems to have been the guiding touchstone for Doug's sadhana, although he also believes in the importance of yoga guides and teachers. "I think it's possible for every-body to cultivate sadhana by themselves, but I think we all need a catalyst to make it happen. It's like you get up in the morning and maybe you don't feel so good and you're kind of negative. Then a sunbeam comes through the window and touches your face and you hear birds singing and you go, 'Ah, yeah.' So it's like the little sunbeam is the yoga teacher that touched you in one way or another, and all of a sudden you're running off on your own."

Doug still recommends keeping a healthy sense of curiosity about your practice. "It's like your parents; you get to an age where you think, 'Well maybe everything my parents say isn't exactly right, so maybe I'll just look at it like this.' You see the same thing in yoga with yoga teachers. You're obedient, you do as you're told and it seems like they must know everything but every now and then you'll think, 'Well maybe I'll try this, or try that.' I think it's human nature to buy into having one diet, one religion, one guru, one type of car. It's easier to just pick one and say, 'That's where I'm going, that's my image, that's my place in life.' It's a little easier for me because I travel so much. I pass through a lot of people's lives, and I view and observe, whereas other people are rooted into a lifestyle, a family, a certain kind of car and a house and a clothing style and a style of yoga. For me it's in constant flux."

My own experience of completing a traditional personal yoga practice outdoors is somewhat limited. I live in the suburbs of a Canadian city where for at least half the year the temperature can potentially be twenty below zero or lower. With a lack of foliage in newer neighborhoods, I'm basically too shy to go out and practice in my backyard in full view of my neighbor sitting on his deck. I also have three young children, and, for me, privacy in an enclosed space for a yoga practice or simply just to sit is a luxury.

However, I have had unique experiences when I have been able to practice yoga outside. While at a friend's cabin recently, I practiced outside on the deck before everyone rose for the day. While meditating one morning, I heard a noise I recognized. When I opened my eyes, a hummingbird was hovering over my head. It stayed for a short while, watching from one angle and then another, before flying away. I also run, and while on longer runs I have had moments when I felt completely connected with the nature around me, when I could not only connect with but also felt that I could draw on the energy of the river, grass, trees, and flowers that I ran beside. There's also something undeniably pleasant about placing your bare feet in lush soft grass or fine soft sand.

For Doug, there is no distinction between inside and outside nature. "I don't really differentiate now between inside and outside. I find it easier to get in what I call 'the zone' when I can hear birds, hear the wind, and have fresh air because even in a sacred yoga studio, there might be paint on the walls and dead trees on the floor and plastic. You might live in Los Angeles alongside the freeway and breathe car exhaust fumes while doing yoga, but you could put a plant in your room. It really depends on you and what connects you. Some people like to have little sacred altars with things that remind them of the path they are trying to pursue. For me, it's easier outside unless it's extremely cold or clouded or there are lots of bugs; then I just compromise and try to bring nature into the room."

Doug believes that while yoga might help us to develop our sense of self, we also affect the environments we inhabit. "I don't like to use the word 'enlightenment.' I use the word 'awareness.' To me, the goal of yoga is to become aware and to know. A lot of people don't know what they want. They get up every day and follow other people around. They say the programmed response and work the jobs they think they're supposed to work and set an image they think will be appropriate in other people's eyes. To me awareness is finding out what it is you really want.

"A more metaphorical image would be like throwing a rock in a quiet pond and it creates ripples and the ripples expand to touch the distant shore. You go 'splash,' and your life is gone, but you create ripples in time with what you say, what you do, how you speak, and what you represent. A lot of people are just thinking about me, me, me. I'm going to get this far and get this house. To me, yoga is something that gives you a tool to realize that your life matters. It's wonderful to have a good time and enjoy your life but within the spectrum of knowing that everything has repercussions, positive or negative things which you leave behind."

While his yoga practice has had a deep effect on the direction of Doug's life so far and the choices he has made, the benefits of his practice are felt on many levels. "I'm sixty years old, and I can still hike and surf and run and do things that little kids can do physically. Mentally, I have awareness that I tend to make better decisions than when I didn't do yoga. Spiritually, I feel a connection with everything."

Yet Doug has also discovered that while the great thing is that he's more sensitive and aware, the downside sometimes has been that he's more sensitive and aware, even if it's leading in the end to making better choices in regard to his well-being. "It is hard to be completely natural and at peace and at the same time fit into a modern, fast-paced, computer-age society. Physically, if you are very healthy, you can smell a cigarette from miles away, and if you eat bad food, you get sick. Mentally, things bother you where they won't bother other people. It's kind of like that saying 'Ignorance is bliss.' When you recognize something feels negative, you wish you didn't know sometimes."

Ultimately, Doug perceives yoga as being a gift in his life, and when he or others for whatever reason might struggle with getting to the mat or in "the zone," he recommends remembering to see sadhana that way: as a gift. "Instead of thinking of it as work, just think that you have this wonderful gift, this opportunity to use your awareness everyday to help expand your life. That's how I think of sadhana; you get up, you can breathe again, and you go out and make the best of your day."

Doug Swenson and his brother David are well known throughout the yoga world both individually and for being brothers, and while talking with Doug, it occurred to me that his sadhana has almost been like a sibling to him. It has been with him in one sense or another since his childhood and, like a sibling, sadhana also has the ability to point out your flaws and perhaps aspects of your being that you can or should change but will also remind you of your good points. Sadhana and siblings not only understand you but also help you at times to understand yourself a little better, and if you're lucky, they will also support you and be there throughout your life: in the moments of life's extremes when we might feel true joy, challenge, disappointment, love, fear, and success and, more important, during the in-between times too.

Chapter Seven

Sarahjoy Marsh

Sarahjoy Marsh is the founder of amrita: a sanctuary for yoga in Portland, Oregon, and is also the founder of Living Yoga, a non-profit program that trains volunteers to teach, and facilitates the provision of, yoga classes in addiction treatment centers, prisons, domestic violence shelters, and to homeless youth. A yoga teacher, yoga therapist, and yoga teacher trainer, Sarahjoy also runs international yoga retreats and service excursions to Third World countries. Sarahjoy also specializes in therapeutic rehabilitation through yoga and in helping women to address addiction and body-centered self-hatred.

When you're in Sarahjoy's presence, you sense there's a thoughtful reason or meditated purpose behind and for everything that she does, every word she utters, every sentiment she shares, and every move she makes. That mindful intent is in her nature. Social justice is a central source of inspiration and motivation for Sarahjoy and has remained a key focus in her life throughout more than twenty years of meditation and yoga practice. "My commitment to yoga as a tool for social justice, through each of us as individuals, has not wavered. The practice of waking up is a constant in all the ways in which I have practiced yoga asana and yoga tools. The possibility of us waking up to our interconnected responsibility on the planet led me to study transpersonal counseling in graduate school rather than basic counseling or social work. It's also where the organization Living Yoga came from. My personal, you could call it, compulsion for social justice is so big that it could have been art for social justice, it could have been gardening for social justice, but ultimately the best tool for me was through offering yoga classes. It's our personal responsibility to wake up, to see our communal circumstances and to be of service in some way. That yoga awakens Living Yoga students to see themselves in this web is super critical. We aren't just changing people by offering these marginalized students yoga; the change is also how they see themselves, and how others have come to see them too. Yoga is a powerful tool for this transformation because of its mind/body connection, and because of its ability to shift how we see ourselves and each other."

Reverence for nature, both for her own and her environment, is inherently linked to Sarahjoy's sadhana, and her yoga journey began as a journey into nature. "When I got out of graduate school, I went backpacking and hitchhiking by myself around the country. Meditation became a lived experience at the Canyon de Chelly, the Painted Desert and in Yosemite Valley. It became a lived experience of awe. I was totally captivated by the felt experience of what meditation teachers had been saying to me for four years. I'd been to many silent retreats by then because I went on them religiously in graduate school. I didn't go on any yoga retreats. I didn't even know they existed, and I probably couldn't have afforded them. But I went to these meditation retreats, and when I was backpacking and hitchhiking around the country, I experienced a felt sense of meditation as living in that awe and joy and connectedness, to nature and timelessness and God.

"That was a pretty big tipping point for me; it completely changed my life. In fact, I didn't go back home. I moved to a retreat center. First I moved to Orcas Island, Washington to live and work at Doe Bay Resort. I was there for one year, and then I moved to Breitenbush Hot Springs Retreat Center in Oregon. I was there for four years. I took a day of silence every week, and I had daily time for yoga and meditation. But I also had extraordinary amounts of daily time in nature and a daily experience of a hot tub and a cold plunge. The experience of the deep rush in your body when you go from the hot tub to the cold plunge is that the mind is totally silenced by the glacier-fed river and there's this incredible experience of timeless expansion. It's powerfully prayerful. There was this huge expanse of space and feeling."

Sarahjoy's appreciation for nature became interconnected with her day-to-day way of being. "At that time I did not have a formal yoga teacher or a formal meditation teacher, because I lived off the grid. So, nature was my teacher, and it was totally profound. In both of the retreat centers, I didn't drive; we walked from one building to the next, and we were constantly outdoors. We had to walk across the river to get to work. Every day you felt the air on your skin, and you could tell when the fall had come before it was on the calendar. You could feel the changing of the light of spring. It wasn't a sudden, 'Oh it's 8 p.m. and it's still light outside. I'm just noticing it now.' You knew it intrinsically, viscerally. I do think that ultimately yoga is trying to return us to our intimate relationship with nature so we recognize ourselves as an expression of nature, not a being trying to overcome nature or the natural tendencies of the body or the heart or consciousness. Nature's a really big influence for me in my practice."

This connection to nature is interwoven into Sarahjoy's sadhana on every level, and she takes into account every aspect of her natural state of being in her approach to her yoga practice. "I do think of sadhana, its definition, as a personal practice—a time on our own, an intuitive or felt sense of what our practice needs to be—and because I'm strongly influenced by Ayurveda as a lifestyle, when I say intuitive or felt sense of what our practice ought to be, it's based on our constitution, our tendencies, our imbalances, and what's happening seasonally as well as what time of day we practice, what the environment is like in which we practice. The entire spectrum is considered in how I put together a home practice for myself or for my students. I think of it as a very critical time for having a touchstone with our deepest purpose, our deepest sense of center. It's not just a chance to fill the gas tank and then go on driving your life. For me, it's really more like you're on a hike and you step off the path to a scenic turnout. There's a really great view there, and you stop and take in the perspective of where you are right then. If we look at it as just filling the gas tank, then we go back to driving our familiar road maps in day-to-day life. We go back to driving in our familiar patterns. I think of yoga as a time where we are researching ourselves for discovery, yes for renewal, but also for discovery about how we wear ourselves down and why we do it and to harness some learning out of that. We aren't just going to our yoga mat to fill the gas tank; we're going for that scenic turnout of discovery and inquiry. It's then necessary to integrate what we've discovered into our daily life, so our whole life becomes a yoga, and the time on our yoga mat is like a sacrament to that."

Being mindful of how we cultivate our mindfulness might seem a little abstract. Yet Sarahjoy believes in the importance of being sure that you are giving your body what it needs to promote well-being on every level as best you can, as opposed to going through the motions of a rote system of sadhana in the same way you might consume a daily multivitamin. "When I say 'scenic turnout,' I mean it's a time to step off the path. So if you're hiking uphill or you're hiking downhill or you've got some kind of goal in mind, it's a time when you step off of that process and you're really inquiring into the nature of your health, at every level, your vitality, and your purpose. Sometimes in a scenic turnout, we discover that we've been driving too hard or in the wrong direction. People might encounter things like moments of sadness, or grief, or moments of overwhelming fatigue that they didn't know were there, or the experience of deep contentment that can be both unfamiliar because of life's busy-ness and yet deeply familiar because of who we are at our essence. I find that if we just stop to fill up the gas tank, if that's what your yoga practice is for, you actually miss those nuances, and that's unfortunate.

"If your life is really out of balance, in whatever way a person would define that, and you find that yoga is 'saving your life' each time you come to your yoga mat, if you're using it to save your life like you would use medication to overcome a headache or to manage menstrual cramps or to block out some other kind of pain or anxiety, I would say stop: because the process of using yoga to medicate your life allows you to keep having a life that's out of balance. The tricky thing here is that yoga *is* medicine, but it's not meant to be medication in the way Americans take medication. So I recommend to my students if they are living a life that is so out of balance that their yoga is only a medication of sorts and it just restores them enough that they can keep going, then what's happening is that they don't have to examine the underlying reason why their life is so out of balance. It can keep the drive going, or it can keep perpetuating the imbalances."

Consideration of time of day, season, Ayurvedic dosha or constitution, weather, experience, environment, and need are inherent to Sarahjoy's personal yoga practice. While both her sadhana and her dharma are intrinsically interwoven, her application of yoga "tools" is both comprehensive and attentive. "My personal practice is a reflection of all of my yoga training as well as what I learned in studying transpersonal counseling. Ayurveda is also a big influence in my personal practice. Additionally, a serious car accident leading to two major hip surgeries definitely impacts my practice, and I don't mean just my physical practice. I mean it's impacted how I approach the practice, based on my more immediate access to the vital body when my physical body couldn't move.

"I had a total hip replacement, and my legs were strapped down to my bed for a few days. I was unable to actually move. You can withstand that for a certain amount of time, and then if you just stay restless in your physical body, you can become pretty agitated. For me, the vital body underneath that was very important. I have studied with physical therapists in a pretty profound way, and they have really influenced my practice. All these streams together, as well as my personal love for the mystical traditions in the world religions—all those rivers feed the ocean of my practice. I'm only nine months out from my last hip surgery. The strongest influences in my personal practice right now are Ayurveda, but for the first three months post-op, the biggest influence was physical therapy. My structural body needed very careful attention and asana at that time."

So how do we best determine whether we are applying our own yoga tools appropriately? How can other practitioners of yoga come to distinguish between applying yogic "tools" in a therapeutic way or simply popping a "yoga pill"? For Sarahjoy, yoga is the answer: a connection to the subtle energies in the body that tell you what you need. "It's like when you go to see a doctor who's really intuitive, and they take your pulses and they read your tongue, like a Chinese medicine doctor. They're offering you medicine based on you uniquely as your own self and what's out of balance with you. When we have a yoga teacher in our lives, it's my hope that the teacher is helping the student to internalize that process. When we go to our yoga mat, we're taking our own pulse. We're reading our constitution and trying to get very sensitive to what's occurring so that we use the practice for medicinal purposes.

"It does take getting quiet enough to hear ourselves. It's a quality of sensitivity that you come to on your yoga mat. It's also a quality of radical honesty with yourself about the minutes and the hours and the days off your yoga mat so you can feel what your life is producing. This is like a kaleidoscope; you turn the kaleidoscope, and the gems are the same, but the perspective keeps changing. If people can feel in their day-to-day life, with sensitivity, how they're running on their energy or their vitality and they can really be accountable to that and sensitive to it, I think we will know intimately if we're going for the medication or the medicine in the practice. When we medicate something, we usually end up with a fairly superficial experience of it, so I think the depth of our understanding is going to be one way that we know if we're in the self-medicating or medicinal use of yoga."

There is a compassionate sweetness both to Sarahjoy's messages and to her voice, and in her classes that I have attended, students seem to be drawn to her energy like a beacon of joy. When Sarahjoy teaches, she often shares tales drawn from her own experiences, like the story of waking up in India to the sounds of monks chanting punctured by the noise of a rhythmic distant tapping. When she ventured outside, Sarahjoy discovered a woman in the act of knocking down the rubble remains of a wall with a small hammer, simply chipping away at it, having faith that the accumulation of her small yet repetitive efforts would completely change the shape of the solid structure she worked on.

Sarahjoy considers that type of faith in the "bigger-picture" intent of sadhana is key, especially on a day when a yoga practice feels like it's somewhat cut short or lacking. "Every touchstone I think is important. When we get to the mat and feel those ten minutes are awkward or not as connected or more uncomfortable, those are the symptoms that are the results of what I call the 'experiments' we were running the day before, or the week before that. If we were overworking or overindulging, and get to the yoga mat and think, 'Oh, it's not what I wanted it to be right now,' well, the symptoms are right there—those are our signals and our information. So I never see it as a waste of time because we're always basically getting results in the form of symptoms and signals and information. When they used to send Morse code, it took a long time for the Morse code to get through sometimes. Some days it's like that for people on their yoga mat, and they don't know what message is coming through. There's an urge to try to guess it before the whole Morse code's been finished. Other days it's like text message; it's right there, and you know what the message is."

The view that how our body is functioning and how we are feeling is the direct result of prior choices or behaviors is, in Sarahjoy's view, a benefit of the sadhana path. "Yoga is defined in some ways as a science. In the practice of yoga, we are the scientist; we're running the research experiments. We're also the thing we're experimenting on, and we are the outcome of our experiments. We're all of those things. So if you look at yoga as your life, the experiment you're running is how you've scheduled your life, how you run your life, how you think, how you act, how you feel, how you behave, the responsibilities you take on or don't take on. That entire experiment is like your yoga, and every day we run the experiment, and at the end of every day or intermittently throughout the day, we see the results of our experiment. We see grouchiness or equanimity, we see fatigue or contentment, we see vitality that's sustainable, or we see fluctuations of mood. Every day we're studying ourselves.

"For me, that is the larger yoga, seeing my actions have results, my experiments have results. Sadhana for me is not just the time on our yoga mat; it's that whole experiment. At the same time, when we're on our yoga mat, we are running a very important experiment. Let's say you practice six sun salutations and four deep breaths and five minutes of loving-kindness meditation and it has a certain outcome. If we're practicing the same thing every day, the practice is consistent, and we are the fluctuation. We get to see, 'How does that practice change me day to day?' I would call that a more beginning-level practice."

Sarahjoy finds that this approach to practice can also change over time. "Once we have a deep relationship to ourselves, what's not fluctuating is consciousness, and we can see how to fine-tune our practice to come back to that ground that is what the *Yoga Sutras* call the place where the fluctuations cease: the second yoga sutra. I think there's a time for using sadhana on the mat where it's a very consistent structured practice so that we get stabilized; we get to see ourselves through the lens of that practice. And then I hope students mature into a season in their practice where they are intuiting based on all they know about themselves. Consciousness is that place that we all know."

A yoga student's cultivation and maintenance of a personal practice is crucial to his or her yoga journey in Sarahjoy's experience. While teachers can support and expand our practice, ultimately it is us as individuals who decide which "medicine" to take. As she explains, "It's really critically important to have a home practice even if you're a regular student at a yoga center. The teacher is coming to teach a class for the group, and we certainly learn something from every class we take, but the practice isn't always tailored to individuals in the classroom. A student can take public classes as a complement to their home practice. Having a teacher is a place for feedback, but the teacher's role from my perspective should be to awaken the inner knowing, the inner intuition of the student, so that when she or he is on their yoga mat at home, they will feel their own voice coming through, not just their teacher's."

Being mindful of your choice of, and participation in, a yoga class is also key to becoming more self-aware or, more specifically, more awakened. Sarahjoy advises being clear on why you might be choosing or avoiding certain yoga classes. "I think a class can be a hindrance because if we take the personality of the student into mind, and let's say that they're of a particular competitive bent, and they go to a class and that stimulates their competitiveness and they go home and practice to come back and be better at the competition, that's a detriment in my opinion. If we're going to yoga class to capture a yoga pose as one might any other material object, I think it's a detriment."

However, even when consciously certain of a mindful participation in both personal practice and group yoga class practice, it is simply the nature of life that challenges may occur. Sarahjoy has faced her own tests in life, but she welcomes them as part of her greater sadhana. "I would say the biggest challenge for me were two very big episodes of heartbreak in which going to my yoga mat meant feeling the level of grief that a human being can feel in heartbreak, in devastation and despair. Those were personal heartbreaks that I certainly leveraged a lot of learning and discovering through, as is my inclination to do so with all my life events. But at the time of the most intense pain in my heart and the sadness and grief, that was the absolutely most difficult time to go to my yoga mat, because it meant encountering that sorrow. Sometimes my body ached terribly with that sorrow, more terribly than my hip pain after my accident, and sometimes my anxiety was so huge, I didn't recognize myself."

Yet this led to Sarahjoy developing an even greater sympathy for other people's suffering. "I felt such wider and wider circles of empathy for people who experience heartbreak, depression, devastation, and anxiety in an ongoing way, because this was a season for me, a three- or four-month season of that. I knew that it was seasonal. I knew it would come to an end, even though I wanted it to end sooner. I had enough perspective and maturity to see it in the larger web of my life. But I felt huge empathy for those who don't have that perspective and who don't have 'swimming skills.' Yoga was definitely one of my swimming skills, yet it was extremely difficult. If I'd had a rigid, structured practice, I probably could have used my practice to dissociate. That wouldn't have been very helpful, and it would have hindered my ability for actually harnessing the experience of heartbreak for my own. I longed for structure then, but I knew it wouldn't serve me as well as simply just feeling.

"One of those seasons of heartbreak coincided with my hip surgery, so I was tied to my bed while having heartbreak; that's pretty powerful. I could have handled hip surgery by itself; that would have been a lot easier, but hip surgery with heartbreak was pretty overwhelming at times. I had a personal mantra to choose love, not fear; it wasn't just my hip surgery that was promoting so much awareness and earnestness and vulnerability. It was heartbreak compounded on top of that."

Sarahjoy has found that a personal practice can be both a therapeutic and a safe place to process emotional pain, to bring balance to both our emotional and physical body, and to learn how to face suffering. "If people don't acknowledge that it's happening or they don't invite it in, it will be prolonged. Our base resistance to feeling that much devastation makes it go longer and feel like it's going to be more deadly. Much like asana, we have to warm up to emotional discomfort. That's where I see the yoga asana practice as a really great tool to teach ourselves how to get comfortable being uncomfortable, how to warm up to our distress, get more intimate with it, how to sense out our limits and our capacities and respond so we have a more rhythmic relationship to our discomfort and our distress and our joy and our capacity. If we use the asana practice in this way and see it as cultivating the tools we need when we're off our yoga mat, when it comes to life, we go out with a tool kit into the world that's pretty incredible. Mindfulness, nonreactivity, distress tolerance and self-accountability—all those things we're learning right there in the asana."

Similarly, Sarahjoy does not see her physical hatha practice of yoga as separate from her karma practice. As in nature, everything has to be in a harmonious balance for the system to thrive, and Sarahjoy recommends ensuring that a practice of karma yoga is serving both ourselves and others as best it can. "I don't separate karma yoga from hatha yoga in terms of yoga for me nor in terms of my daily sadhana. There is daily service to others, and it's not my paid service. It's another service to others where we lessen our sense of self-absorbedness, the unhelpful kind of self-absorbedness, and we increase our sense of interconnection with others. However, there is a time to pull back, when what we're doing is causing an imbalance. If a person takes on a karma yoga practice and they take it on with a particular lack of maturity about it, that could lead to a pretty fast road to burnout. If how they interpret karma yoga is serve, serve, serve, it's all selfless service, serve to God, give it all over to God, surrender, surrender, surrender, and they're not maintaining the reservoir out of which their service comes, then I would say to them,

'Stop serving.' If the serving is underneath a level of self-interest that keeps getting generated and that's causing an imbalance, I would say, 'Yes, stop. Stop the imbalance that you're creating.'

"With a hatha yoga practice at home, a person's personal asana practice, if it's become rigid and hard and a place for self-criticism or condemnation or of white-knuckling it through your life, I would say, 'Yes, stop.' But in all cases, I would say, 'Stop and feel the pain that you're actually in that generates these decisions to produce these actions.' Our ability to stop and feel the pain that we're in can be learned through both karma yoga and hatha yoga. In karma yoga, we learn it when we feel the pain that someone else is in and let it awaken us to our own pain, not harden us to it, not fix their pain but awaken to our own. In hatha yoga, we practice awakening to that pain when we feel the hamstrings or the shoulder blade or a particular ache in the heart with heartbreak. But our willingness to stop and feel the pain that we're in in this country, in this culture, is abysmally low, so we keep generating more ways to avoid that pain and discomfort. There is a time to rebalance your sadhana: I would certainly say take a look at that, examine it."

This explanation and example of asana offering more than purely exercise to the body can open a realm of possibilities in terms of what your practice can be. In my own experience, the realization that my asana practice didn't have to look like physical exercise was a huge relief. Sarahjoy explains that while exercise has its benefits, your yoga practice will benefit from being a distinct time spent apart from a workout. "I am a bike commuter. Every day I have my daily practice for asana, pranayama, meditation, and I ride my bike to and from my yoga studio. I differentiate them in that my exercise is specifically functional. I'm going to raise my heart rate and increase my circulation. It's wonderful that my bike commuting is outdoors; I'm in the elements, I'm in the community, I'm in the traffic, and I'm in the flow of life. My asana, pranayama, and meditation practices are more internal, and it's like a little refuge or retreat."

Similarly, Sarahjoy finds a more formal practice of yoga can offer a sense of sanctuary. "When I do my home practice, I'm stepping away from the world as we see it on the outside, but I'm stepping into the world of nature as me, as this expression, this body temperature, this heart rate, this muscle's movement, this synapse that makes it happen. I'm stepping into the world of consciousness, but I'm stepping out of the material world for a while and the world of my responsibilities. It is a tune-up, it's a renewal, yes, but more than that, it's prayer, gratitude, giving thanks, and opening myself to vitality so I can serve others."

Attending to that recalibration and sense of openness and appreciation does at times take discipline. Sarahjoy has strived to honor that devotional commitment wherever she might be and welcomes both the good and the bad sadhana experiences as processes of progress. "When I was backpacking around the country, my consistent 'location' was that I had the same blanket that I was traveling with from one place to the next. The actual geographic location changed, but the physical ritual of that blanket was important to me. That was a representation of my practice, I ritualized that piece."

Over the years Sarahjoy's practice has come to have more of a regular routine time and location. "I do have a dedicated yoga space in my home now; I practice when I wake up in the morning, and I have a consistent wake-up time. When I'm traveling, I keep that same routine. When I'm teaching a retreat, often I have to break up my personal practice between asana and pranayama and meditation because the retreat has a 7 a.m. class. I have part of my practice before I teach and then part while the students are having breakfast. It does fluctuate when I'm teaching a retreat, but because it's been so consistent for so long and I have a dedicated space and dedicated time, it's easy to stay with it. It's much like you wouldn't consider not drinking a glass of water each day. Some people wouldn't consider not showering. I've gone a day without showering, but I wouldn't go a day without practice of some kind."

How that practice might look, however, is suited to Sarahjoy's needs and circumstance at that moment. "Lying in my hospital bed, my practice was reading Pema Chodron's *When Things Fall Apart*, giving thanks for the nurses and a Tonglen practice for all those who were also suffering. Because I had a complication after my surgery, my practice was also feeling how profoundly vulnerable my body was. I lost too much blood in the surgery, so part of my practice was feeling how awful my body could feel and just being in awe of that. I didn't want it to stay that way, but that was the reality. I think people mistake progress in yoga as progress in asana. There are several poses that I will never do again because of my hip replacement, that's totally fine with me. I smile upon the opportunity to have these limitations."

Sarahjoy's innate sweetness extends to her viewpoint on what might be considered the "dessert" of our yoga practice: savasana. Occasionally, students, seeming to perceive that their yoga "work" is done, will roll up their mat before they get to feel the outcomes and results of their efforts. Sarahjoy feels strongly that savasana is not a course to be skipped. "Savasana is a time of integration, and as such it should not be excluded. You've just shaken the salad dressing. Let it sit on the counter; it all settles. The spell you feel from savasana is so critical; it's like getting the antenna hooked up to God. I'd rather have my antenna functioning than not."

For Sarahjoy this kind of connection comes naturally. "There's a constancy in my life, and it's having the antenna hooked up to God. Even though I have my moments of irritability or frustration or overwhelm, there's a constancy for love and service. My yoga practice reminds me of that every day, it's like a communion with that every day. My yoga practice will also tell me when I'm too busy. The thought, 'I don't have time for a full hour this morning' or 'I don't have time for that much,' is a good reflection that I got overscheduled. My practice can yellow-flag my attention rather than waiting for a red flag."

When I recall the times I have felt connected with nature, when I have paused for a moment and placed my bare feet on summer grass or soft sand or in a mountain stream and simply taken a deep breath, the memory is very potent and real. In that moment, I have felt all that I hope to gain from yoga: a connection with peace, the divine, the universe, nature, my body, my mind, my spirit, my emotions, everything. While the effects of that feeling may not have lasted for a whole hike, or a whole afternoon at the beach, or even a quick coffee break in my own garden, in that instant, everything was good. Similarly, Sarahjoy explains, moments on our mat are not to be judged or dismissed either. "I would say, overwhelmingly, it's really important not to come to your mat with a self-critical voice. Honor every effort that you make to get to your mat. Cherish every time you're able to be there and let the feeling of your yoga haunt you enough that it magnetically pulls you back when you go off course. I don't think that criticism is a good motivator generally, but that magnetic pull of what yoga has offered us can pull us back again and again."

There's a reason we are drawn to nature, to want to walk in a park, or on the beach, or through a forest. In the same way, surely, taking time to connect with the nature of ourselves helps us all to grow.

Chapter Eight

Erich Schiffmann

Erich Schiffmann is the author of *Yoga: The Spirit And Practice Of Moving Into Stillness* and has created numerous DVDs, both those with an instructional asana-based focus and also those with a more philosophical and spiritual emphasis, including *Freedom Style Yoga*, *Moving into Stillness Workshop*, *The Wave and the Ocean*, the *Erich Schiffmann Backyard Series*, and *Erich Schiffmann at the Feathered Pipe Ranch*. Erich has also produced the downloadable recording *Spokane Yoga Workshop 2010* and the guided meditation CD and app *iMeditate with Erich*. As well as providing workshops and teacher training, Erich continues to teach regular yoga classes at a center in Venice, California.

As part of the process of completing this book, transcripts were typed of all the interviews, and as the project progressed and the reviewing and editing were completed, there was one specific term that came up over and over throughout each and every conversation: "you know." It may be idiom or slang, but in this context perhaps it's more than a simple slip of the tongue or a coincidence. The statement that was uttered during all the conversations about practicing sadhana was *you know*. If there is a proponent of this approach in terms of his teachings and exemplified practice, then Erich Schiffmann would certainly be a contender for that title.

Erich was drawn to yoga in his high school years through reading about Eastern religion, spirituality, and meditation. He has studied with many teachers including Krishnamurti, Desikachar, Dona Holleman, and Iyengar, resulting in decades of personal yoga practice. The focus of Erich's sadhana now is on listening inwardly for guidance and validation, and he aims to help his students to do the same for themselves. "When I teach a normal class now, in chapter one, I talk for about twenty minutes, and people have questions. In chapter two, we meditate together for between eight and ten minutes. For new people that seems like a long time. For someone who is more experienced, it seems really short, but it is a good amount of time. In chapter three, I guide people through the poses. At that point they're learning to listen to the human teacher—me—and override their conditioning about things. Chapter Four has become this free-form chapter, and when I first started doing it, it was very short. I would say something like, 'Class is almost over, but if there is another pose or two that you would like to do before sliding into savasana, take the next minute and do exactly what you feel like doing.' That's how I started the free-form chapter. People liked it. Everyone could think of one pose to do or if they wanted to get a head start on savasana, they would. Then I started playing music, and it lasted for one song and then for one really long song, and at this point, that chapter's about twenty minutes."

To some it may see a little unconventional, or one might perhaps even feel duped in going to a class and paying to spend part of the duration directing your own practice, but providing a context and environment for a self-guided practice to unfold and nurturing how to make that connection is at the core of what Erich aims to share. "The free-form chapter is me no longer telling anyone what to do. What I tell them to do is listen inwardly for what they feel like doing in a roomful of other yogis doing the same thing. At first there was resistance to doing this, but once it clicked and once people got it, they really started enjoying and preferring finally being given the freedom to do what their energy is feeling like doing. Now that people know that there is a free-form chapter at the end, and at that point they can do exactly what they want to do, people listen to the human teacher's instruction more than they used to during the human teacher chapter, which again helps them override their conditioning."

Though there were instances of resistance, Erich persisted in his teaching. "I remember somebody said, 'I'm paying for this?' I was explaining what we were about to do; I wasn't going to give instruction for a few minutes. I wasn't going to walk around the class and give adjustments. In fact, I was just up there at the front of the room doing my practice. It felt like it would be a higher teaching if I was actually doing the same thing with everybody instead of me walking around the room adjusting everybody. It feels like we are finally flinging into what the real sadhana is about: being 'online' and listening for what to do. Then being free enough to give expression to what you find yourself knowing when you are listening like that and doing it in a safe context with other yogis who are doing the same thing. You start to get the hang of how to do your practice and how to listen."

This idea of tuning in to a greater teacher inside was elemental to Erich's exposure and study of yoga from the beginning and was an aspect of his attraction to a personal practice. "I remember liking the idea, that there was such a thing as sadhana. That there was a lineage of experience behind people's practice and what to do to be clear on all of this. I was also raised around Krishnamurti, and he was sort of known as the 'anti-guru guru.' His teachings were to not follow anybody's teachings, and so there is a subliminal put-down of sadhana in a sense. Yet he was only saying that because the true sadhana is self-inspired."

While one might perceive that being directed to listen to an internal source of guidance by an external teacher can seem a little contradictory, Erich explains how this approach to yoga worked for him. "I think the rare individual can get along without guidance, but someone who is doing that is actually in touch with real guidance. All the teachings essentially are to help you get to the place where you are online all the time by yourself. In a sense you become your own best teacher, but in a truer sense, you realize that you are not your own best teacher, but you have found a way to hook into, or connect in with, the real teacher. So it feels like you are online and you're in learning mode all the time. To other people it looks like you are your own best teacher because you are not going to classes anymore. Yet really you know that you're not your own best teacher, but you've learned to listen essentially."

On reflection, Erich finds that it is also the discipline of sadhana that has led to freedom on many levels for him. "As I look back at what happened to me, and what's still happening to me, I was with Krishnamurti, I was with Iyengar, Desikachar, I met Krishnamacharya, and I was interested in what they were all saying and when my sadhana kicked in, I was being very structured in what I was doing. I was taking others' advice, and I liked having it all mapped out because basically I didn't know what to do. I was getting advice from people who had learned from other people who had learned from other people. This was centuries of advice being hand-delivered basically. I was happy there was advice to follow, and I was very good at being structured and disciplined about it."

However, for Erich, the discipline itself led to unexpected sadhana challenges. "For a lot of years, on Monday I would do this practice, on Tuesday I would do this practice, on Wednesday I would do this practice. The whole week was mapped out essentially, and I liked that for a lot of years. After about ten years of that, I started not enjoying my practice, and I found myself rebelling against the discipline. It felt like everything was going wrong. In retrospect, I realized that all the discipline, all the hard work, was working. After many years of the disciplined structured practice, the discipline was actually working in the sense of if the structure works, it will start to dissolve. The discipline, the structure, builds sensitivity. Then once the sensitivity has been cultivated, the energy starts taking over. You don't just do back bends because it's Wednesday. Instead, you start transcending the discipline, start transcending the structure, and you start trusting your inner sense about what to do or not do.

"That was a real confusing time for me because no one in my world was talking about transcending the structure or going to the next level. It was still about, 'Do the discipline, do the structure, do what the teacher says,' whereas if you do all that, and if it works, the structure and the discipline will begin to dissolve. Then you'll start surfing your sadhana in a technique-free way, which is sort of what Krishnamurti was trying to say, but I wasn't really getting it. I found it very helpful to have the structure. Prescribed practices can be very helpful, but the implied meaning should be that if you do the practices, they will build your strength, build your sensitivity, increase your ability to transcend the discipline. If you don't discipline yourself, the tendency is to just act out whatever you've been conditioned to do. The discipline helps you override your conditioning so you don't just keep doing the discipline; you start flowing with the movement of the life energy. Which is the point actually: not to just be good repeaters of discipline but to actually be sensitive humans living life."

Yet letting go of a discipline, a style of practicing yoga, or making a change isn't always easy; the truth isn't always kind. Erich found that seeking out a new environment for both himself and his practice helped to literally shift things. "It was a hard period for about two years because my whole understanding was undergoing transformation and this sort of earthquake and tsunami in my mind. Things were getting shaken up. I wasn't enjoying the practice, I wasn't enjoying going to classes. I was still teaching because I had to make a living, but I was feeling conflicted about what I was teaching. Basically, I moved to a new area and got into new surroundings and stopped going to classes. I just stayed home and did my own practice and gradually began to clarify what was happening. It felt like things were really going wrong. I couldn't have kept doing it the way I was doing it and have success with it or have fulfillment with it—it had to push me out of itself in order for the new growth to occur."

An overall affection for the feeling of yoga sustained an underlying connection and motivation unswayed by doubt that kept Erich from breaking his relationship with yoga altogether. "I had been so in love with the subject for so many years, and then I started to not be in love with it. I didn't like the feeling of not being in love with it. That feeling started to come back, and so that was the clue: 'Wow, I am starting to enjoy this again; life is starting to make more sense again.' I started feeling inspired again instead of tired. Instead of doing the discipline just because that was what I was told, I started feeling the life of life again, and it felt really good to feel alive again. I finally realized that the training was what helped me get to this point, so I wasn't upset with the teachers or the practices once I realized they were working."

Maintaining a teaching practice helped Erich sustain his sadhana. As he explains, "I've been making my living doing this. I never did it to just pay the bills, but if I wasn't teaching, there certainly would have been bigger chunks of time where I probably wouldn't have done anything. The fact that I was teaching is good because it kept me in the game. Otherwise, who knows, I may have just dumped the whole thing. I can't really imagine that, but because I was teaching, it helped me."

Yet Erich sees sadhana as something greater than a practice of yoga tactics. "The practice essentially is not so much how you bend over or how much asana you do but what you are doing with your mind. The easy way to talk about it is using your mind to be online. Not everyone likes the computer Internet analogy, but it's just an analogy. I like it because it actually describes yoga in a very succinct way. The word 'yoga' means 'yoke,' it means 'to join.' When you join, you feel your unity. 'Yoga' means 'yoke,' and it means 'joining' and 'union,' so it is very much like the Internet except bigger. You are using your mind to join with 'Big Mind;' your mind to join with the supreme. When you join with the supreme or you use your mind to get online, you start to get the sense that this 'Big Mind' that you are getting online with *is* your mind, like you only exist because the Totality of things is erupting as you. When you use your mind to get online, finally you find that you have a bigger perspective about things than you had previously.

"The real sadhana is to then live your life with the perspective that you find yourself having when you are online. The idea I have been pushing the most lately—and it seems like the yoga world needs to be refreshed with—is that yoga is a lifestyle. It's not just a sadhana that you do as a portion of your life. It is actually the Totality of how you do your thing. The essence of it is always listening, listening, listening. Whenever you need to know something you ask 'Big Mind.' You get online, and then you learn to silent mind it for half a second even. When you silent mind it and you quiet your mind, the download flows in, and you find yourself knowing whatever you needed to know. Be attentive to what you are doing with the mind and use your mind to be online and listen, all the time, to the best of your ability.

"I remember talking about it with friends, and they asked, 'Why would you want to silent mind it? Why would you want to be in a thought-free state? It sounds moronic. It sounds like the opposite of what you want to do.' But what happens is that when you are able to silent mind it, better knowing comes in, better answers come in. It is not moronic. Actually you find yourself being a little smarter than you were a moment ago. It is extremely life affirming."

In the beginning however, while Erich was attracted to yoga, his process of developing a personal practice at times required discipline. "I was drawn to it, so that took me to the yoga mat, but there were certainly aspects that were difficult. It took me probably six or seven years before my personal practice actually kicked in. I was trying to do it, but I would go into the room and think, 'Maybe I should go wash the dishes' or 'Maybe I'll go vacuum the house'; suddenly all these other things seemed more appealing. I had difficulty actually establishing the practice. I was trying and I finally realized that listening to other people's advice helped me know what to do, so there was less confusion about what to practice or why. I just wish at some point someone had said, 'Well if you really get into this and you follow the teachings, they will finally culminate in a free-form or a freestyle practice.'"

With this hindsight, Erich relates the practice of yoga as bringing a freedom of self-expression similar to how other activities that require practice can result in masterful self-expression. "I am not familiar with jazz music really, but the idea of it is that you learn how to play your instrument, you learn how to get good at the notes and the scales, get good at all the 'stuff,' all the discipline, but the real point of it is then to get in touch with music and start improvising and letting your skilled practice bring out the music. If someone had just said that, then I would have gotten into the strict practices knowing that you are doing this in order, in a sense, to create your own style.

"I grew up in California, everyone here surfs and goes to the beach and I had surfing idols. It was sort of understood that a good surfer was someone who came up with their own style, their own unique expression of it. They would do a similar turn to somebody else, but they would put their little own flare on it. If someone had just said the whole point is to be the human that you are, not just a copycat, but learn all the 'stuff' and then put your own unique self-expression on it, then I would have embraced the discipline. I would have done the practices but with the knowing that they culminate in something beyond just the discipline."

Erich came to that conclusion on his yoga path, but his journey did not culminate at that point. He continues to practice regularly, getting online to determine and meet his personal practice needs. "I do it on a need-to basis, but it does turn out to be every day. My schedule is pretty free, so my practice is to be online listening for what to do. Rather than going into the room at 6 a.m. until 7:30, now the discipline is to be listening for the right moment. The time changes, but I usually go into the yoga room about 5 p.m. I like it late in the day; I have done my day, and I then give myself more permission to go into the yoga room and be there for as long as I want because I have done everything I have needed to do. When I'm in the room, I've got my notebook, I've got my laptop, I've got my tape recorder. I'm doing my practice, but I'm also writing. I'm also listening for insights. It's just a fun learning mode time. I'm not making myself do anything especially, not like I used to. What I'm doing now is always listening for what seems to be the right thing to be doing."

At the time of writing this book, Erich has been practicing yoga for well over forty years. When he pauses to calculate the actual number, even he himself is surprised. "I have had a lot of practice with the practice. I started when I was fourteen, so whatever that is. . .forty-four years. . .whoa. . .forty-four years. That is a lot of time to get familiar with what works for me and what doesn't work. Part of it is the amount of time, which I guess is the same as getting older."

While there may be an observed correlation between a maturing of sadhana as a person grows older and more experienced, there are still core aspects of Erich's personal practice that have not changed in almost five decades of practice. "The thing that hasn't changed is I'm still learning. It feels fun to be involved in something where the learning hasn't stopped. It actually feels like I am getting better and better at learning, and part of what yoga is about is always learning."

While Erich is continuously listening internally for insight, that does not mean that his more traditional realization of a personal yoga practice is always completed alone. In fact, Erich often practices with friends and advises that there are times when this might help other yoga practitioners too. "If someone is having difficulty practicing, I would suggest that they invite some friends over and do free-form together. A couple of times a week, friends of mine come over, and we practice together. I'm in the room from 5 to 8 p.m. People just come over for as long as they can, or they leave when they need to. The room's not real big, so there can't be very many people, but people are always coming in and out. We're all just doing our free-form practice. I'm not leading it, and people are doing their own thing. It's totally fun. Sometimes I'd really rather just be in there by myself, but it is also really fun practicing with other people."

Having a space to retreat to by himself or to gather with friends and share a yoga practice is appreciated by Erich, who hasn't always been blessed with a space within his home set aside for the exclusive purpose of yoga. "I haven't always had a space; that has made it difficult. I would highly recommend, if you can, have a space that is just waiting for you, that really makes it easier. Even if you use the room for other things, at least it's there calling you; that really helps. I think basically do anything that helps. Often I will put music on because it helps me get into it. Just be free enough to use whatever seems to increase your ability to participate in doing the practice. The more you practice, what you find helpful will start to shift and change, but increasingly you figure out what works for you and just keep doing whatever seems to be working. I used to put on the Rolling Stones a lot, non-yoga music, but it motivated me; it got me going, and I like that."

In terms of determining whether we need to draw on external sources of sadhana motivation or whether the practice we are striving to commit ourselves to isn't suitable for us, Erich recommends looking at your experience of joy on a day-to-day basis as a trustworthy gauge of whether you are treading along the right path. "I think the sign it is right is if you find your life increasingly interesting; life seems worthwhile. Whereas, if you are living in a way that you are not enjoying your life, then do your best to change it. For example, when I first got into all of this, I was very strict about diet, I was a strict vegetarian, but after a lot of years, I started finding my energy wasn't what I had hoped it would be. At that point it caused me to reevaluate. I didn't like doing the right things and then not feeling the payoff. I realized that I've just got to do whatever helps me feel excited about life because otherwise it feels like I am just doing time. I want to feel excited about life and enjoy life, so I changed my mind about what was important, and at that point I started listening to inner guidance for what to do. It's not as easy as it sounds but let go and to the best of your ability ask 'Big Mind,' 'What should I eat right now?' Silent mind it and then just be attentive about what sort of foods pop up into your mind and then eat them."

While it may seem that taking time to make more mindful choices or completing a traditional yoga practice may result in momentarily withdrawing from life, Erich has found that consciously connecting or being online results in him being more present and aware and more thoroughly living his life moment to moment. "In a sense you've got to step away from the chaos in order to slide into your peace to the best of your ability. You're stepping into life with the practice. You are actually participating in a better way. It makes you a better human. Life goes better; somehow life reconfigures, and things just seem to flow better when you're doing this. You do get external validation from the world that you're on the right track, whereas if you were doing this and everything was always going wrong, it would alert any semiconscious person that what you are doing might not work.

"It is so self-life affirming, actually, not antilife. It's not just going along with the way it's always been. It's like sinking below your conditioning and getting in touch with the life of life so you're moving away from old ways of being in order to get in touch with the true new movement. I think for a long time I just wanted to get enlightened so I could get out of here, whereas actually it's here; just be here and see what's going on differently than how you used to see it. That is sort of the idea that I think, in the yoga world, needs to be refreshed: of getting gaga about life again, getting impressed with how awesome life is and then trusting into it, trusting into yourself because you are the specific expression of life. By trusting your deepest impulses, you're actually evidencing your faith in the movement of life. I think that is good."

For Erich, this introspective style of guidance is spiritual in essence. "Getting online and listening for what to do is the same as 'Thy will be done,' so I don't think it is in conflict with any of the religions that I am aware of. Yoga is not a religion, but it sure does induce religious feeling. The word 'religion' means 'relink,' which is almost identical to the word 'yoga,' 'to yoke, rejoin,' and I like that. I think it can actually enhance whatever anyone's religion is rather than conflict with it."

What Erich considers the best sadhana advice he has ever received is short, sweet, and easy to remember: he was directed simply to "persist." Having steadfastly applied this ideal to his personal yoga practice, the reward has been that it has brought more truthfulness to his day-to-day being and actions. Similarly, the sometimes challenging consequence of that is his practice has brought more truthfulness to his day-to-day being and actions. As Erich explains, "My personal practice is to be online, and what's hard about that is that some of the time it will encourage you to move in ways that you don't always want to move in, encourage you to do stuff that you may not want to do. It makes sense why it would work like that because you are getting in touch with the supreme consciousness and you start desiring to have that guide you. It is going to guide you out of your littleness, and there is going to be resistance to moving beyond your little comfort zone. So, as much as you want divine guidance, at the same time there is likely to be resistance to it. You will be guided to do stuff you don't want to do. You'll be guided to make phone calls or go on workshops that you think you don't want to go on. The first step is realizing that you want 'Big Mind's' guidance, and the second is being willing to embody it when you start hearing it. It's not that easy always, and sometimes you think the guidance you get conflicts with family members, but increasingly you realize that whatever guidance you are getting is taking the whole picture into account. I find it easier and easier to go with the guidance flow, but it will move you in ways that you think you don't want to move in. You don't have to do it, but then you suffer the consequences basically."

While listening to guidance might not always lead you along the easiest path, Erich has found the positive results of his actions provide a validity that inspires him to keep checking in with his internal moral compass, an action that he finds increasingly easier to do via means of meditation as opposed to other available yogic tools. "I am less interested in the contortionist aspect, whereas before, that used to be really high on the list. When I was a kid, I had a manual toothbrush, and I would scrub. Then they came up with electric toothbrushes, and I would do that, and those worked better. Then they came up with sonic toothbrushes, and now those work better. It seems like in a similar way, it's possible to get the same benefits that I was trying to get through the physical practice, actually just through meditating. The more online I am, the more there is no dissonance in my field that I need to work out, or there's less. I can conceive of the time where I wouldn't need to bend over at all, where I could just sit and meditate and suddenly be clear. It would be faster and better, but I'm not at that point. I still have the desire to move and stretch and erase tension by doing that, so I do, but I am doing less."

Erich has found that by quieting his mind, getting online, and living in a more truthful capacity, he is more himself: he is living life *more*. "Trusting yourself is what it comes down to, and it makes sense to trust yourself because you are the Totality in specific and unique self-expression. Mostly we've learned to not trust ourselves, but sadhana is about getting us back to the place that it makes ultimate sense to trust yourself. The important thing is to sink into your deepest impulses; those are trustworthy. If you don't trust yourself, it's such a weird predicament to find yourself in. What do you trust at that point? It finally comes around to trusting yourself, and it makes sense because who you are is the Totality. You are not just trusting your conditioning, but you are trusting the deeper force which is erupting as you. The discipline, the structure, the practices are about helping you be you better, not trying to become something other than you—not changing yourself so much that you are not recognizable to yourself anymore but becoming the true you—not getting rid of yourself, just being a better expression of the Totality."

For Erich, the result of trusting in himself and connecting with internal direction has not only brought a greater gratitude to his way of living but has also consequently brought more joy. "All this takes you to the place where you start appreciating life more. You start walking around being wowed by life more. You start naturally feeling good inside because the energy is good. It's so soothing to finally feel the deepest, truest truth about who you are is loveliness. The truest truth about life is loveliness. The truest truth about anybody is loveliness. Life isn't the enemy; you can trust yourself. There is an intelligence to things. Therefore, let go of what you think you know, sink into your deepest knowing and silent mind it, and then dare to do what you are being guided to do at that point. It's sort of an easy formula. It gets easier and easier to do but is pretty advanced. I feel optimistic about things. The world's not going down the tubes; it's reconfiguring. You end up feeling naturally optimistic. You start believing in love. You start believing in intelligence. You start believing in wisdom as being the source of what's going on. It feels good."

Chapter Nine

Robin Rothenberg

I would like to pre-empt my next sentence by saying that Robin Rothenberg is not old enough to be my mother, and neither does she look like she could be. However, from almost the instant I met her, I felt like I was being "mothered," not in a patronizing, condescending way but in the sense that I knew I was in good hands—I knew I could trust the lessons and learning that she offered. You can tell pretty quickly that Robin has vidya and avidya down to a fine art and that she can see though your avidya for the both of you. That's how she's like a mother—there's love, without doubt, but there's also an element of tough love, of truth, of hitting home, or showing you how to hit your home for yourself.

Robin was certified in Iyengar yoga through 1996 and is a certified Viniyoga Therapist. For twenty years, Robin owned The Yoga Barn studios outside Seattle, and she now focuses on teaching therapeutic yoga within medical settings. A member of the advisory board of the International Association of Yoga Therapists, Robin was also an adjunct faculty member of the yoga therapy certification program at Mount Royal University in Canada for four years. Robin facilitates yoga teacher and yoga therapist training programs as well as international retreats and workshops. Robin has also developed *The Essential Low Back Program* training and CD/book set, the *Soothing the Spirit: Yoga Nidra to Reduce Anxiety* CD and facilitated the *Living Yoga Radio* talk show, which is available on podcast. Robin also continues to see private clients and to offer group therapeutic yoga classes.

Robin has been practicing yoga for over a quarter of a century, and interestingly this began almost immediately after the birth of her second child, who was born in close succession to her elder sister. As Robin's yoga experience has grown, so her daughters have also grown. As Robin recalls, "From the very outset of my exposure to yoga and my journey into it as a student, there was this idea of practice, that one practices, one has a sadhana. I didn't necessarily understand what that would look like, but I knew that there was that expectation that if I didn't somehow learn how to do that, I wouldn't really be a yoga 'practitioner.' I knew that that was an underlying requirement, and early on I didn't have a clue as to how to get that really up and going. I went to classes, but I didn't really know what personal practice meant for me.

"Then I had a deep revelatory or epiphany kind of experience of growing a personal practice organically, which for me happened in that first year that I started taking classes. I felt so great after my class, and then through the course of my week I would end up moving back into my malaise of chronic aches and pains and health issues. I remember one day realizing at some point that the baby was sleeping, my older daughter was occupied with coloring, dinner was on the stove, my husband wasn't home, there was nothing I had to do for anyone else for a minute, and I remember thinking, 'Downward dog would feel so good right now.' I remember doing it, and nobody cried. I didn't get in trouble, and I thought, 'I could do another pose.' Then it occurred to me that that was how my yoga practice needed to be at that time in my life. As a new mother of very young children, I was on call but it was up to me to take note of the moments where I wasn't needed and to take care of myself in those moments."

This dedication to claiming yoga for herself and development of a person-al practice, albeit in fleeting quiet moments in a busy day, was the beginning of a journey that affected not only Robin but her family too. The positivity that Robin generated in her practice was tangible to the point that her chil-dren and husband could clearly tell when she had or hadn't practiced because of the impact it had on their lives. "I remember there was a time when the girls were maybe six and eight and I'd been snarly with them about some petty thing and they said, "Mommy… don't you want to go do some yoga now?' My reaction was, 'Ah, it's important that I practice, not just for me, but for them.' I got it, it was a hygiene thing, like 'Don't you want to go brush your teeth?' or 'Really, you need a shower, Mom.' They didn't know what I did in that room, but they knew when I came out, I was nicer; I was a more pleasant mommy.

"Up to that point, the question was, 'Am I being selfish by taking time for my practice?' That by focusing on me somehow I was taking away from family time or delaying the time when we could all go out together because we had to wait until Mom was done with her practice. None of this has anything to do with them; this was all my own sense of personal guilt I was carrying. When they said that, it really gave me permission to step fully in and say, 'This is important for me; it's important for our family that I do this and take care of myself.' It's no different than getting the right food, than getting the right amount of sleep, than taking medicine if I'm ill. It really helps me to be a more calm, more clear, more open, balanced, healthier person on every level when I do my practice."

A question of guilt is something I'm sure a lot of parents can relate to, as can anyone who feels like they have other obligations they could be attending to other than practicing yoga. For myself, I know without a doubt I am a kinder, more compassionate person and, more importantly, mother, when I have had a chance to complete my practice or even to attend to it in some way. I often joke that luckily each time I gave birth my head didn't fall off; I can participate in a conversation beyond the realm of diapers, tantrums, and homemade baby food. I also know that I do need to connect and remember the whole "me" to fulfill my role as a mother the best I can; otherwise, I feel like the person whose whole reason for existing is to empty dishwashers and pick up underpants. There's a value to that, obviously (who wants to trip over unwashed underpants?), but I don't think I'm going out on a limb by stating that I think most of us yearn for more depth in our daily lives. That may be where I am in my sadhana journey. I still need my personal practice of connection to remember myself. However, while guilt was once an issue, I have learnt to let it go.

Robin empathizes, "My husband traveled a lot when the girls were young, so I was the sole caretaker for them a lot of the time. Then when he was home on the weekends, it was our rare family time, so I would feel bad if I wasn't being family oriented, but he was always really supportive. He would say, 'Go do it. I'm home now.' So often times, it was just my own issue. Yoga has helped me through that and I'm less encumbered by that kind of stuff and I see how I held myself back by believing a lot of things that weren't even true. My girls now have a really good sense of knowing when they need to take time out for themselves, whether it is to take a walk or just have some time alone. I feel like my modeling the importance of sadhana was actually one of the best parenting gifts that I gave them. I modeled for them that it was okay to take time out for oneself, that I wasn't available 24/7 to be a mommy machine, and that mommies need to be replenished. I discovered for me what replenishes me is yoga practice while encouraging them to find that which is nourishing to them."

Just as children have many key developmental markers—learning to crawl, walk, and talk or their first day of school—similarly there can be key milestones or feelings of positive progression in the development of a personal practice. Having nurtured a personal practice for over twenty-five years, Robin has come to a place of loving gratitude and compassion toward herself and her practice and again feels a clear link between the people who are part of her life and her sadhana. "I have been married for thirty-one years, and I have been practicing yoga for twenty-five years, and I have a similar experience at this point with both, which is some days it's good, some days not so good. It doesn't matter; you just show up the next day, do not get too concerned. Sometimes I'll come to practice, and I'll feel really distracted, and I'll have a lot of trouble really focusing my mind and I'm aware there's a level of agitation. I don't judge it like it's a bad practice; it's just a reflection of my state of mind. It helps me to understand what I'm bringing out into the world and to ask myself about what's going on underneath it all.

"Likewise, sometimes with my husband, we're totally in sync, and sometimes it's like we're speaking completely different languages, and I think, 'How in the heck have we managed to raise two children and now a granddaughter?' I don't judge us or him as harshly as I used to. Now I see it more as that's just how it is today. It's a continuum, and there's no question that I'm going to show up tomorrow and love him and support him and support our family as we grow old together, and there's no question about whether I am going to practice tomorrow; it's just part of my life. Some days I feel like I never want to get off the mat, I feel like I just want the practice to keep unfolding and unfolding, and other times I think, 'I don't have any time to practice. How am I going to practice today?' Then I decide, 'Okay, ten minutes, go, make the most of it.' It's a whole different kind of experience, but I still show up. Sometimes I literally unroll the mat, stand and take five or ten breaths, do uttanasana, sit down, say a prayer, connect, and that's all I have time for, but it's better than not having any time. There are days that that's all I have time for in my relationship with my husband. It's like we're going in opposite directions, but I say, 'I have you in my arms right now, let me look in your eyes and say I really love you. Okay, have a nice day, bye!' "

One of my first yoga teachers used to refer to time that you might have spent doing yoga being redirected, sometimes unexpectedly, toward your children or family responsibilities as "family yoga," a term that has helped me immensely, especially during moments when I have to miss that yoga class I really like *again*. Yes, being a parent always comes first, and that kind of responsibility doesn't come without its sacrifices and challenges, but these are also opportunities to grow, and that translates to my experience of yoga when I feel like I am participating in more of a conscious practice off my mat.

Robin can relate, and she has also come to appreciate the benefits that a change in sadhana perspective can bring. "I would say there are times after I have taken an intensive training or I've been giving an intensive training and really been immersed in yoga that I might say, 'You know what? My sadhana today is to focus on the yoga of relationships or the yoga in my garden,' to put my attention elsewhere, to give it a breather for a day, maybe two.

"Just recently my husband and I were in Thailand visiting our daughter, and I intentionally didn't do a practice. I gave myself permission to not focus on it. Usually when we travel, I always have my yoga mat, which I actually did bring, I never leave home without it, but we were in a variety of different locations, and I didn't trip out about missing my practice. If I felt the need to practice, I would practice a little. I don't have any recollection of a really deep, strong practice for those two weeks, and it was very refreshing. It was the first time I stepped back from it, and I felt really good the whole time.

"When I came back, I was so aware of how much my energy had been outwardly focused. It felt yummy to come back home inside, to set my mat out as my little sanctuary to reconnect to my heart, to my soul, to my mind and my body and say my prayers and breathe, do my pranayama, and to move with that sense of just where and how my body wanted and needed to move and just be really internally focused. Distance makes the heart grow fonder. Like a love affair, it was just natural. It was the right thing for me to be there with everybody doing the schedule like that, and then it was really nice to come home to my routine and reconnect."

However, for Robin her sadhana isn't something that just makes her feel good. The effects of not practicing and thus not feeling *as* good helped bring her to her mat. "On the physical level I have many years of experience of feeling dreadful and then getting on the mat and doing something, anything, and feeling better. My husband used to hand me the keys and my purse and kick me out the door and say, 'You're going to class.' I'd come home and he'd say, 'How do you feel?' I'd say, 'I'm fine, I feel great, why?' not even remembering how bad I felt before."

I think I have asked more questions of Robin than of any other teacher I have taken yoga training with. She was the first teacher I ever approached during a break in training, and it was because Robin had expressed passionate views around the topic of yoga and exercise. Robin maintains a clear point of view on the two. "My body actually needs exercise to be healthy. I have areas that hurt if I don't exercise regularly, so I'm actually a big proponent of exercise. Our bodies were meant to move and meant to be lived in. To use asana as the only form of exercise, the only form of feeding the annamaya kosha, is a disservice on many levels. I can spend thirty minutes on my elliptical, break out in a huge sweat, get my heart rate up, and never do that in two hours of asana. I have a very busy, full life, and so I think, like most people, I have to be efficient with my time and energy.

"Yoga and asana are not synonymous. I think asana is beautiful in orientation. However, if we're trying to use asana alone for exercise it's not efficient. If I go for a walk up the hill with my dogs, not only do I get outside in the fresh air, I do something good for the dogs as well. If I go on the elliptical and get my heart really pumped up for thirty minutes then I'm free to take my yoga practice time to develop more of a meditative process of connection. I can use the asana to tend to and care for the parts of my physical body that need tending to that haven't been addressed through exercise. I can work with my breath, my vital energy, my mind, and touch into places emotionally that allow me to connect to God."

While it may not be exercise, Robin finds that sadhana can contribute toward health and well-being on many levels. "People are so fragmented. Everybody's busy, everybody's running around crazy, feeling frenetic, feeling rushed, everybody's running late, on their cell phones, text messaging. To have the time to get still and to tune in instead of tuning out, to collect ourselves and to breathe, just to feel our own being, it's not just a gift, it is a gift *and* it's a necessity for sanity. We need something that helps us to get back inside and to ground ourselves. We need it for ourselves, we need it for our family and our community. We need it for our world because in a world of people who are 'meshugana,' that's a Yiddish word meaning 'chaos,' we're crashing into each other and creating more messes. Whether it's being a better mother or being a better wife or being a better coworker, a better boss, whatever, to be more grounded inside of ourselves, we all need sadhana. Yoga happens to offer so much in terms of the shape and variation on the theme of sadhana that there's something in there for everybody. Whether it's a purely physical practice, a breathing practice, a meditation practice, a mantra practice, a visualization practice, deep relaxation, study, introspection, or reflection, there are so many tools, but they all lead us back home to our own heart and soul, which is where we gather our energy. If it's all dispersed, then what we have to offer is really fragmented; it's not coming from a solid core."

On the topic of yoga teachers having a personal yoga practice, Robin's passion for sadhana surfaces still more. "This is my bias, and I feel comfortable making this strong statement: If you're going to step up and say that you're a yoga teacher, you need to have a personal practice. If you're not practicing regularly, you have no business teaching yoga. It's unethical to not have a practice, and that practice can be study, it can be meditation, it doesn't have to be an asana practice. However, if you're teaching asana, it's important to stay tuned in to your physical being and to observe changes as you grow, as you age, so that you can have that more readily available to share with your students. But definitely you need to have some kind of meditative practice that's connecting you to your heart, to your soul, to the teachings, and to God, to Spirit, to divinity, to that which is greater than your own little ego-self."

Part of that connecting with and living in truth can lead us to moments of change. To begin with, Robin exclusively practiced Iyengar yoga, and then, as her practice progressed, she began to be drawn toward other traditions of yoga, namely, Viniyoga. "When I practiced Iyengar yoga, I never thought outside of the box. There was a right way to do things, and I always tried to match what my teachers had told me. Then when I started studying with Gary Kraftsow and studying Viniyoga, there was a whole different set of rules, some in direct opposition to the rules that I had learned through Iyengar yoga, so there was an unlearning, and a relearning process. I found myself at times feeling torn between two lovers. For the first several years that I studied with Gary, I really just immersed myself in the Viniyoga tradition and the sequencing principles, which I actually hold true to, to really come to understand that tradition in and of itself. I found, once I had a good handle on that, that some of the teachings from the Iyengar tradition were filtering in. I realized, although a lot of that fell away, there were pieces that never fell away. I started owning it and saying, 'Oh, this is true for me. It has nothing to do with what the teacher says. This, in my body mind complex, really works.' Since then, I have been exposed to a variety of other non-yoga traditions. I've gone full circle, from doing only what the teacher told me to, now I trust my own experience. On a particular day, it may look very Iyengar, or it could look very Viniyoga. On many other days, it wouldn't look like any one thing, it would look like some kind of amalgamation."

The benefits of this evolution and self-prescribed method of personal practice have been profound for Robin. Through it she nurtures and maintains a better connection to herself, to her family, and to a greater divine energy. "My health continues to sustain, emotionally I'm more balanced, and I get into less conflicts with people in my life. I feel more open in my heart, softer, more receptive, and less defensive in general, so I'm more open to criticism or feedback from family or other members in my communities. I credit any positive developmental signs in the way in which I am in the world to my personal practice without a doubt. I do feel like the feedback I get from my husband and my children, in particular, who are the people who have to spend the most time with me in close quarters, that I'm easier to live with is a good thing. I feel lighter at heart. I feel more forgiving of the people who may have hurt me, and I feel a deeper connection to my own spirit, soul, and to God, and all of that feels like evolution."

There is a Jewish proverb that states, "God couldn't be everywhere, so he created mothers," and for as much as being a mother and practicing yoga is part of Robin's life, so too is spirituality. Over the years, Robin has found that her personal yoga practice and study has served to support her spiritual development. "I am Jewish, and I'm very connected to my Jewish heritage, not just culturally but also religiously. I spent the last two years in a Jewish spiritual direction training, which has brought me more in touch with the mystical, spiritual teachings as opposed to just the rituals of holidays and services. What I discovered is that everything that I've learned and loved in the yoga teachings about what it means to develop one's soul and spirit and become more aligned, more ethical, more compassionate and tolerant, it's all in Judaism. When I study the Buddhist teachings, and I've been exposed to a lot of the Christian texts too, it's all the same: how to be a good person, a caring person, a contributing person for the welfare of others and how to get outside of our own ego, need-based perspective to look out in the world and say, 'How can I contribute to the good and the well-being of the world as a whole?' Yoga's about becoming more whole with ourselves, and the holy is held within the whole. Part of becoming whole within ourselves is really connecting with our spiritual self, our soul, and so the holy is within the whole of our being; it's all one."

This sense of openness and acceptance extends to Robin's sadhana, with Robin being open to whatever might arise as her personal yoga journey continues to unfold. "My mat is now a canvas and I just come to it empty. I bring my body, I bring my heart, I bring my soul and I bring my breath. Then I lie and explore the wholeness in my being. I have this great tool chest that is really big and deep, thanks to my wonderful teachers, and my understanding of myself that has grown over the years through my yoga practice. How I apply those tools on any given day has to do first with my sitting and con- necting. I feel blessed, and I say thank you literally every day for all of my teachers because they're always with me on the mat and informing me. The ingredients that go into a cake, cookies, bread, or pancakes are all basically the same. The outcome is dependent on how those ingredients are mixed together. By altering the amounts of each ingredient, one can create an end- less variety of flavor and texture. My practice is like that too. There are the same basic ingredients; there's usually some asana, there's always pranaya- ma, meditation, prayer, mantra sometimes, but which ones and how they're combined has to be decided in the moment based on who I am. I love practice, I love sadhana, and I hope I continue to grow and learn about myself as well as the power of these tools so that I can share that with others forever. It's endless, it's infinite." Just like a mother's love.

Chapter Ten

Leslie Kaminoff

Leslie Kaminoff's *Yoga Anatomy* book has found its way onto the shelves and into the hands of hundreds of thousands of North American yoga teachers and students. Inspired by the tradition of T.K.V. Desikachar, Leslie is the founder of The Breathing Project, Inc. an educational non-profit dedicated to providing advanced studies programs for movement professionals. Leslie offers international and online courses, workshops related to yoga, anatomy, and breath and continues to provide private yoga sessions. Since 1998 he has also facilitated the online list and blog, *e-Sutra*.

When I first started attending yoga classes and then began yoga teacher training, it seemed that I saw Leslie's book everywhere—for sale on yoga studio shelves, on recommended reading lists, in the hands of many teachers and fellow students, for sale at conferences—but it wasn't until I heard him speak at a conference that I finally bought it. When everyone tells me something is good, defiantly, I tend to resist it. A little stubborn, yes; stupid, at times, perhaps; but it doesn't matter either way: I like to learn my own way, to experience a lesson for myself. It turns out that so does Leslie.

"Pretty early on in life, I extracted myself from structured learning environments. I was never much good at school. I learned to read and write but beyond that I really did not function well in classrooms. I later came to realize this was because I had some learning disabilities, a certain type of dyslexia, which I only discovered when I was in the midst of writing *Yoga Anatomy*. I barely got out of high school, then spent one semester at a very liberal unstructured college, which was still too structured for me. I started living and working on my own at the age of nineteen in New York City. I was very fortunate to have had the support early on from my parents as I found my own way. What I eventually connected with and was passionate about turned out to be yoga."

I think it was also fortunate perhaps that Leslie had the confidence to make the choices that he did. When I first saw Leslie at a yoga conference, he was simply an energy to behold, and I mean that in a very positive way. There's a confidence he radiates, a definite sense of being sure of himself and of his own nature of being and what he's doing. Not in an arrogant way—he just seems full of an awareness of life, and it is reflected in his vitality. Ultimately for Leslie, breath is everything, and his connection to it and his embodiment of it results in a vibrant presence. Leslie's connection to yoga was forged at the age of twenty, after experiencing just one yoga class. "The one thing I remember specifically from my very first yoga class was the immense shift that occurred in the final relaxation. It was the first time in my life I entered into a state of conscious, intentional relaxation that didn't involve falling asleep. It was really a revelation to me and I wanted more."

For someone who might typically avoid structured classes and group learning settings, it is surprising that Leslie's attraction to yoga led him to register in a six week beginner's class at New York City's Sivananda Center, coincidentally now only a couple of blocks away from The Breathing Project. "I believe the first time I heard the word 'sadhana' mentioned or defined was in the context of that beginner's course. There are two major books of Sivananda's: *Sadhana* and *Bliss Divine*, and they are both very, very imposing and intimidating. I think some of my initial negative reactions to the idea of sadhana originated when we had all of this material thrown at us: if you want to be spiritual you need to do this, this, this, and this, like the japa, the mantra meditation, the purification, the right thinking, the right living, the right diet, all of these things. Perhaps because the usual context for sadhana is spiritual, it took a long time for me to actually get around to understanding that a literal translation of the Sanskrit is simply 'a means of accomplishing something.' "

Leslie continued his commitment to being a student of yoga and strove to process the immense sadhana-related resources and information for himself. This eventually led him to become a swami and work within the Sivananda organization. "I went to India with the Sivananda organization, took sannyas, came back a swami – I was very much steeped in that whole tradition. I was young enough that it really did inform my growth and development all through my twenties. In a way, it was those sadhana practices – on my mat at a regular time, with certain intention – that structured my growth and development, not just as a yoga educator but as a human being. It continues to be part of me, how I carry myself through my life, how I relate to gravity and to my own breath and thoughts. It informs everything I do."

Although there seems to have been a choice to follow the path of yoga, Leslie's innate confidence and connected awareness of what is right for him laid the foundation of both his life course and his life work. "This is the only career I've ever had and most of what I do each day is directly related to yoga. In addition to teaching it, I try to exemplify yoga in my interactions with people, whether students, coworkers or clients." Leslie's dedication to sadhana and a yogic path led to a conscious breath-centered way of being and the founding of his New York-based organization, The Breathing Project, Inc., as well as moment-to-moment realization of what he experiences as spirituality.

"The root of the word spirit is from the Latin 'spiritus' – meaning 'breath.' When I met Desikachar in 1987, he transformed this whole relationship I had to my breath, which I had been cultivating for nine years prior to that, and it was enormously transformational – and very disturbing, in the beginning. If you ask me now what is my regular spiritual practice, it's that: focused, intentional breathing work with other human beings. It's not confined to the hour-long segments I divide my workday into, where the client work fits. It's also when I'm just relating to people in general, whether the people I work with or those I teach or my family.

"In Malcolm Gladwell's book *Outliers*, Gladwell writes that if you want to become very good at something, the minimum number of hours you need to practice is about 10,000. I found that very interesting and did a conservative calculation in my head of how many hours I had spent doing individual one-on-one work with people. It was well over 20,000 hours! That is a lot of time to spend consciously breathing with other human beings, and if that is not a spiritual practice, I don't know what is.

"The breath makes connections – there is an exchange there, a rhythm that varies from person to person. The texture of it is incredibly complex and endlessly fascinating and ultimately enlivening and enlightening, and being involved in this dance on a day-to-day basis is a continual focus of my life."

When I first contacted Leslie about being interviewed for this text, he emailed back that he didn't think that he was the kind of person I would want to interview because he doesn't practice sadhana. Doesn't practice sadhana! I literally read that response just as I was walking out the door to go to a yoga class taught by a friend. When I got to class, guess whose yoga book had inspired and helped shape the class she planned to share and was sitting in her lap? Leslie's. When I told her of the content of the email I had just received, she replied, "What! Now I really want to know what he has to say!" "Me too!" I emphatically agreed.

I recontacted Leslie, and he agreed to be interviewed, and that's when the deeper reality of how his sadhana is inherent within his life became apparent as well as the fact that he uses yoga tools on an "as needed" basis because his sadhana, like his breath, is in every moment. "At this point in my life I throw down the mat and do asana from time to time when I need it, when I feel stiff or something gets hung up or stuck in my body or my life. Asana practice has always been breath-centered but as I get older and stiffer I'll probably have to do more stretching just to live my life and do my job. I don't need to put my leg behind my head now. I don't need to do a ten-minute handstand. I don't feel a burning desire to master the third series of Ashtanga. I do desire to maintain the level of strength and mobility and integration that I require to live my life, playing basketball, riding horses, playing with my kids, being able to demonstrate poses without embarrassing myself in front of a room full of people. I'm not asking for much. As I age, I expect I'll have to do a little bit more work to maintain that, and I'm okay with that."

Although it might change in how it looks as a traditional utilization of the tools of yoga based on need, the "how" of Leslie's sadhana is inherently linked to the breath, just as the "what" he is connecting to or with is essentially the breath also. "I get to observe a lot of people doing something that looks like yoga practice, but the difference between something that looks like yoga practice and actual yoga practice has to do with a deep inner connection forged via the breath between the mind and the body. That's something that happens internally. You can't look at someone practicing and say, 'Oh, they're doing their sadhana.' Their mind could be off in a million directions, and they could just be doing things by rote, unconsciously.

"In the second chapter of Patanjali's *Yoga Sutras*, 'Sadhana Pada,' he describes this tripod, this three-legged support for practice. The first thing he mentions is Tapas. In essence, this means working outside of your habitual tendencies. It's like my teacher T.K.V. Desikachar says, 'Your yoga practice always has to be a little more clever than your habits.' I see no value in doing something by rote, repetitively, day after day. That's not a spiritual practice, it's just habit. I'm not saying it's not useful, but you can do that in a gym. What makes a practice spiritual is something different and deeper and it has to have this quality of Tapas: changing the things in your system that are changeable.

"You also have to recognize that there are things that aren't going to change, and you shouldn't waste energy trying. This is the second leg of the tripod, where Ishvara Pranidhana comes in. It's a deeper concept than simply 'Surrender to the Lord.' I am an atheist, so that concept of surrendering to the Lord has no meaning to me, but I certainly recognize that there are things in my life and universe over which I have no control, and these may be very powerful forces. The question is what sort of relationship I have with those things, and that's where I practice an attitude of surrender. The breath has this dual quality of being both voluntary and involuntary. When you are doing a breath-centered practice, you are confronted with this reality right from the get-go: there is only so much control you have over your breath. This is why, for me, the breath is the ultimate teacher of sadhana.

"The third leg of the tripod is Swadhyaya, represented in my practice as the introspection and self-reflection that allows me to distinguish areas of Tapas from areas of Ishvara Pranidhana. In that sense, my understanding of that sutra is no different from Reinhold Niebuhr's famous 'Serenity Prayer':

having the strength to change the things you can – which is Tapas, the serenity to accept the things you cannot change – which is Ishvara Pranidhana, and the wisdom to know the difference – which is Swadhyaya. This is a universal truth, and it is expressed beautifully by the reality of our human breathing mechanism, both voluntary and involuntary."

I have spoken with atheists, I have spoken with people who consider themselves spiritual, but I have not often spoken with or met people who define themselves as both; they don't typically go hand in hand, not in a confident, consciously, reasoned way. Leslie clarifies how he came to this coherently tangible and cogent belief. "I connect with the thing that makes me take my next breath. I don't have to go any further to find the source of what's keeping me alive, a force far greater and older than I. It's an ancient, ancient thing. All I have to do is pause my breathing and wait – something arises inside of me over which I have no ultimate control, and it makes me take the next breath. It has always been there, it has never not been there. It didn't have to be created, it is the source of creation; it is the causeless cause. I don't have to extrapolate a distinct entity to be that cause because then I would have to ask, 'Well what caused *that* thing?' It's an infinite regress and at a certain point I have to stop asking and accept that causeless cause. The universe that I inhabit, that inhabits me, that moves through me with every breath I take, *is* that causeless cause. There is no need for me to go somewhere else to find the source – it's the thing that's been making me take my next breath ever since I took my first breath.

"When I studied anatomy and embryology in this context, I came upon some very profound truths, like the fact that I had circulation in my earliest forming system right after conception – before there was a heart making it circulate. Where did that movement come from? It's inherited; all of this movement is inherited. I got it from my mother, who got it from her mother, who got it from her mother, and it goes back through every mother, through every womb, through every species that ever reproduced, through every ocean that gave birth to every life form, back to the Big Bang. That is what is moving the blood in my body right now and moving the breath in my system right now, and I can dance with it for a while, I can fool myself into thinking I have some control over it, but that control is very limited."

The idea of there being a will or force other than our own seems overwhelming, awe inspiring, and humbly comforting; we are both significantly insignificant and insignificantly significant. Leslie witnesses these kinds of realizations in people through his work nearly every day. "The leap for most people is understanding and accepting that every breath you take happens because the universe pushes air molecules into your body. All we have to do is make the space and the universe fills it. It may sound simplistic or obvious, but people who have breathing disorders don't get that. They think it's their constant effort that's keeping them breathing, and that's a very stressful universe to live in. As soon as they grasp that the sea of air we live in wants to push itself into their bodies and all they need to do is make space, they shift to a very different and less stressful way of living. I see it happen all the time in the work I do at The Breathing Project. People come to me with severe breathing disorders and we have some really, really good success helping them. It's incredible, and very fulfilling."

Not only being witness to but also being able to offer support and guidance during that kind of change and realization in clients is a privilege that Leslie does not take for granted; for him it is both a spiritual practice and an affirmation of his sadhana. "My ability to sit or stand with these people while this is happening and be present in my body, in my breath and in my attention, that is the fruit of my early training and practices." Although Leslie's lifestyle is an ongoing fulfillment and experience of his sadhana, in the early days of his personal practice there were elements of self-imposed guilt in terms of finding a sadhana rhythm that he had to work through to find a more peaceful way of practice. Fortunately, his own sense of self-awareness helped him become, appropriately, more self-aware. "I used to have a lingering sense of guilt and self-criticism, 'Oh, you should be doing sadhana. Look at all those people, they're doing their practice every day, and blah blah blah.' Now, I know a lot of people who do a lot of yoga practice, and some of them are real assholes. The number of hours spent on your mat has no direct correlation to how good a person you are in the rest of your life. The real question I needed to ask myself was, 'How good a person am I? How do I relate to the people around me and to myself?' I've got a pretty good life and the last thing I need is to guilt myself about not being on my mat often enough."

This gratefulness for his life experiences and opportunities led to Leslie's never really questioning if he was on the right path. "There was never an alternative for me. I'm like a sponge, I absorb by putting myself into environments where the stuff I'm interested in is present so I never really had that question, 'Am I on the right path?' I may have had stray thoughts over the years – 'Why don't you go to medical school?' or, 'Why don't you become a licensed massage therapist?' or, 'Why don't you go back to college?' – but those thoughts would last about two seconds before I'd remember, 'Oh yeah, right, you're *you*. You're the guy that does not function in structured learning environments or learn very well following other people's agendas for learning.' "

Leslie might be acutely perceptively self-aware, but he also comes across as a passionate person, and this zeal for life has sometimes led him, as we all do from time to time, to spread that self a little too thin in the face of appealing opportunities, resulting in our either consciously or unconsciously retreating from the outer world a little to remedy that imbalance. "I think a function of my personality is I tend to over-commit and then the resulting stress makes me want to withdraw, but that's just sort of a rhythm of life that I recognize, having been doing it for the better part of fifty-four years. Fortunately, I am very, very lucky to have gathered an incredible team of colleagues and coworkers and people who have found a home here at The Breathing Project. We're really thriving and it's wonderful to be part of. I just had to get out of my own way and not let my habits get in the way of this incredible thing that's flourishing here."

Again, in either an unconscious or a conscious way, Leslie feels that while his connection to sense of self, to yoga, to his sadhana and the connection that brings to something greater than himself, may have resulted in the creation of The Breathing Project, the opposite is also true. The Breathing Project and the life it contains, maintains, and sustains equally reaffirms and reflects the choices he has made – like an inhale and exhale, the two feeding into each other. Leslie, self-depreciatingly, puts it down to his ego. "My friend Krishna Das' description of his sadhana really hit home for me. He once told me that 'my spiritual practice is my chanting and my singing, and for some people, they can do it alone in a room and be perfectly fulfilled. If you want to get a sense of how stubborn my ego is, consider the fact that I have to do it in front of hundreds of people for it to be my practice.' This helped me realize that though there are some amazing, beautiful, sweet, enlightened, spiritual people who may never appear on the pages of *Yoga Journal* or show up in a Web search or anywhere else, I need to do it differently. People like me are the ones who end up in this book, the really stubborn egos who have to put ourselves out there so thousands of people can remind us of who we really are."

Just as Leslie's sadhana seems to serve him on every level, he advises seeking out a way for your own personal practice of yoga to serve you. "Don't listen to anyone else's ideas about what you should or shouldn't be doing. Find something you connect with, stay connected with it and see where it takes you. Find something you're already connected with, that you're already doing, and figure out a way to deepen it and keep doing it. Sadhana is a means for accomplishing something you want and, for me, what I want is to be more connected. I'm very fortunate to have found this breath-centered orientation to yoga and my teachers, particularly T.K.V. Desikachar. It all keeps pointing back to simplifying and to getting all the extraneous stuff out of the way. That is what the breath is."

Simple.

Chapter Eleven

Ted Grand

On the day I met with Ted Grand, he was moving. He hadn't mentioned this state of affairs—not that it mattered at all. When I arrived at his home, I was very graciously invited inside by his sister-in-law for tea, and we waited together for Ted. He and his family were at that stage of moving where you wish you could clone yourself three times over just to get even half of your to-do list done. Boxes blocked every room and doorway; the move was imminent. Ted's life was on boil, the act of repositioning himself and his family a catalyst bringing about change and progress in his life, the intensity purging away any excess from life, clarifying it to its essentiality. I was sipping tea and chatting with his sister-in-law about yoga when Ted arrived completely on schedule, completely calm and unflustered, even friendly, not a small achievement for anybody when moving.

Ted Grand is a cofounder of Moksha yoga, which is considered to be a style of "hot yoga." Ted also created the sequence of postures of Moksha yoga, drawing on the experience of his own practice as well as his wide range of yoga, yoga teacher and yoga therapy training with many prominent yoga teachers.

However, it was a passion for social justice that originally led Ted to yoga. The idea of yoga providing a way in which to live your life in a balanced way came to Ted almost as a remedy to a life being lived seemingly out of balance. As he explains, "My background, prior to yoga, was environmental activism. I was very involved at university with environmental clubs, outreach, and education, but post-university, I wanted to apply it in the working world. I started off working with Greenpeace and then started becoming more active, working on specific campaigns. As with most NGOs, the more you are successful with something, the more work they give you. The next thing you know, I'm working twelve to fourteen hours a day, blockading logging roads, hanging off of ships, getting arrested. I don't say that so much as a point of curiosity but a descriptor of how everything unfolded. I got more and more angry the more I got involved. As we tend to do in our late teens and early twenties, we want the world changed the way we would like to see it, and we want that change immediately. That's not a very sustainable way of being. In order to force the change, I became more and more radical, and was drinking pretty much every night; it was impossible to maintain that much fire and intensity, and I burned out. I just couldn't sustain that kind of energy, and that's what dropped me into sadhana."

From a life that was spent being not only so outwardly focused but also concerned with the well-being of something as enormous as the Earth, Ted retreated from the outside world and turned his focus to the world within. "What I was trying to do was change all the external variables (the world) without changing myself, and that's what creates that psychological break. Nothing (not even one's self) can match up with the ideal, and thus great suffering is born."

Ted moved to rural British Columbia and began meditating and practicing yoga. "I was living in an old cabin up on the side of a mountain with no electricity, was growing my own food, and had a big old beard - I was almost a cliché of sorts. I practiced on my own in front of this wood-burning stove and with each movement and each day, a sadhana was born. I had a photocopied sheet of a fax of the Bikram series; I had no idea that there was an actual guy named Bikram, I had no idea about the heat, I just did it because it made me feel better. I had no idea there was a system of yoga called Bikram or studios."

Ted considers that his yoga journey began practicing asana in that cabin and that, "it kind of unfolded from there." That unfolding has come to include trainings with many teachers, including Acharya Yoganand Karandikar, Georg Feuerstein, Judith Hanson Lasater, Rod Stryker, John Friend, and Patricia Walden.

Ted also completed yoga teacher training with the founder of Bikram yoga, Bikram Choudhury. However, Ted's beliefs brought about deviations from the traditional Bikram style and with it a sense of conflict. "What we did with Bikram yoga was kind of verging on antithetical to what his approach is. We were doing ecostudios. We weren't following a script, which is required with Bikram, at times modifying the sequence and basically teaching it from a very different perspective. There were complaints from other Bikram studios because we wouldn't put carpet down, for example. He got pretty upset, and I understand it. In his lineage, you do not question your teacher. You do everything that the teacher says."

Ted came to a moment of realization that his situation had to change. "I was at a speaker event where the presenter was talking about living your truth. He said that you can never be part of an organization where you don't feel absolute trust in the person who's leading it. A light went off and I called up Jessica Robertson (co-founder of Moksha Yoga) and said, 'We have to leave Bikram Yoga.'"

Ted's perspective of yoga practice continued to evolve during his yoga therapy training with Dr. Karandikar in Pune, India. "It was at a really cool juncture of my life because you get into your thirties, your body starts to shift, and you can feel a different response to the poses and the sequences that you do. It was at a perfect time for me to study yoga therapy, because that slowing down of the body just wove in perfectly with the perspective of my teacher in Pune (Karandikar). I don't say this as criticism necessarily as much as observation but in Bikram, it is all 'go, go, go'. Part of the dialogue in a standing backward bend, for example, is 'go back, way back, fall back, it's going to hurt, don't worry, it's supposed to hurt!' That's where my head was in this very physical and forceful practice. So to learn what I learned in Pune was earthshaking. It totally reconfigured how I practiced but also set the tone for the creation of Moksha."

However, there were benefits of the Bikram tradition that Ted believed were valuable, as were other elements of his yoga teacher trainings. Ted and his partner decided to ascertain exactly what it was in their yoga experience that seemed to work best. "We decided to take six months, and we analyzed the hell out of it. 'What is the ideal yoga community? What can we do with it? How can we use it as a vehicle for progressive ideologies?' What came out of it was Moksha. There are a few really defining factors which contributed to our vision. One was outreach, trying to make it available to people who wouldn't otherwise be able to do yoga. So we started up karma classes, which are by donation only, and if you don't have the money, you don't pay, with a hundred percent of the money going to charity. We wanted to make it accessible to people who wanted to practice regularly as well, so we instituted an energy exchange program where people do cleaning, accounting, massages, front-desk work, any service that they could provide in exchange for yoga. We went to town on the 'green thing.' We had already been doing ecostudios, but we wanted the peak-most green of the green you can get. Obviously, teaching and the actual asana had to be a part of it. At that point, I had done the two-year program in traditional yoga with Georg Feuerstein and had done yoga therapy training in Pune with Dr. Karandikar, and so we incorporated three aspects: 'How can we honor the traditions outside of the lineage model? How can we incorporate yoga therapy into it? How can we incorporate the best of what we had with Bikram as well?' I guess that's kind of how Moksha came to be."

For me, although typically I don't participate in any kind of hot yoga, in my own personal experience, it's amazing how much the body can "open up" in that kind of environment. I live in a location that not only is very dry but can also be severely cold, as in fifty-below cold (no, I do not live in Antarctica). In the midst of last winter, my family and I escaped to Maui for a week. The day after arriving, when I practiced, the difference in my body was astonishing, to the point where it felt like I had been given a completely different body to work with. The stark contrast of the environmental influences of increased heat and humidity resulted in poses I've never been able to quite manage at home coming easily. By coincidence, there happened to be a short yoga workshop on during the time we were there that I attended and again, the difference in my body was amazing to me. I was doing poses that I didn't honestly think I'd ever do.

Heat is one of the attributes particular to Moksha yoga. Of course, the way in which heat is created and maintained in the Moksha studios is as positively eco-conscious as possible, but the heat itself is considered to be a quality of the practice, not an objective. As Ted clarifies, "I think it's a complement to a practice, but I don't think it defines the practice. Personally I like the physiological response in a heated environment, how the fascia responds and how that allows the muscles to slide. I like the detoxification aspect of it, particularly living in a modern world. I think that's very important. I like the effect it has on the immune system, the digestion. That said, it's not a rule in our community that that's how it has to be. Most all Moksha studios offer some classes that are in a non-heated environment as well."

So, if you're a dedicated Moksha practitioner, a personal practice can be developed outside of the studio without installing an extra furnace in your home or incurring extortionate heating bills. However, I wondered how it feels to have something as personal as a yoga sequence inspired by your own practice become so hugely popular with other people, to the point of repeatedly filling up teacher trainings well in advance. With over seventy studios in North America in operation, and with no signs of the progress or popularity of Moksha yoga slowing down, Ted finds pleasure in watching something like the Moksha community manifest and thrive in a very alive way.

"The irony of it is that I love the chaos. Isn't that funny? I think that the universe tends, and nature tends, towards complexity. It doesn't stay static, and it's always evolving and changing, and I think there's something unbelievably beautiful and sacred about that. The more we try to contain things and create the static state, the more suffering we'll create. So when I see this growth of the community and it taking on characteristics that we might not have set out to create, I think it's beautiful. The more color and character that it develops, even with the pain of growing and changing, I think that's cool, but boy, does it hurt sometimes. I'm in the middle of a move, and there are some struggles involved with that in terms of community and family and sangha and re-creating a lot of things. That said, that's the nature of nature. In nature, things crumble and fall apart too, so if that happens with Moksha, so be it. It will take on new shapes, characteristics, and outlooks, and that is a healthy thing. It may even not be called Moksha Yoga at some point - who knows?"

Though Ted expresses a "letting go" and "non-grasping" take on the Moksha community, he sometimes observes a sense of accumulation playing out in the yoga world. "One of the biggest present-day challenges in the contemporary yoga world is this tendency toward hyper-physicality. It's a very powerful force because it's intimately intertwined with a workout mentality of this kind of consumerist, accumulative approach to asana but also the physical effect. There's nothing wrong with a really strong practice only because the effect often is one of just feeling so alive and so in tune. It would be great if more people could exercise, but if that's your primary focus, then you miss out on the richness of the experience."

However, Ted sees his personal practice as greater than the time he spends on his mat, and he plays down both a sense of accumulation in his sadhana and of hierarchy in the realm of the Moksha world. "We don't set ourselves up in Moksha yoga as a hierarchical or vertical structure. We try and continuously create this horizontal management model. That said, people will want to elevate you. I sometimes feel that pressure of, 'Oh, I've got to keep up with my practice for that reason.' Fortunately the rebel in me always rebels strongly against that. If I miss a day of practice – whatever. If I miss a week of practice, it doesn't matter. I'm so committed to making this about a real way of living in the choices I make with my family, with my parenting, with what I purchase, the food I eat. It's holistic, and it's a full package deal."

Ted believes that it's important to keep your sadhana in balance, including your perception of how it is realized. "It's somewhat important to keep a practice in perspective. I feel strongly about demystifying things, particularly in the yoga context because there is this desire of people to re-create the patterns and intricacies of religion. If you put so much power into one element of your life, in my opinion, it creates imbalance. If it comes down to the asana, I think it's silly. It's about taking a minute out of every hour and breathing, feeling my diaphragm, being really aware of how my body is moving and feeling in moment to moment, and that directs me in the choices I make. So when I'm shopping or when I'm thinking about a kid's birthday party or what kind of car I'm buying or what kind of vote I'm making at voting time, that's the practice."

Similarly, the principal guiding measure of success for both Ted and his business partner Jessica Robertson is a mindful presence of peace. As Ted explains, "We were two years into Moksha yoga, and we were approached by people from an EMBA program at the Ivey School of Business at the University of Western Ontario. They wanted to use Moksha as their case study. They met with us several times, interviewed us, and came up with this overview of what they saw Moksha yoga as being in terms of community but also as a business model. One of the questions on the first survey was, 'Why are you doing what you're doing?' Most of the questions you checked, yes, no, here's what we think, here's what we are, here's what we're wanting to do, but this particular question stumped both Jess, my business partner, and I. We were doing this separately, and both of us answered in one sentence: 'To help create peace in the world.' We always keep going back to that. Whenever we feel there's a lack of peace in our lives, we know that something's wrong with our business model, with our practice, with our communication; that's always the light that's directing our path as a community. If there's a lack of peace, then something's wrong, and trust me, the bigger a community gets, the less peace there tends to be. We make mistakes, studio owners make mistakes, teachers make mistakes, students make mistakes, and it's an unbelievable social experiment we have going on right now."

The personal practice of yoga can be viewed in terms of experimentation. Just as there are times to practice, there are times to assess and reassess the process. Ted believes a teacher can be an intrinsic and objective part of that analysis. "We're very complicated creatures, and we have a lot of nuance that I don't think we're necessarily aware of day to day. I think it's absolutely essential that we come up against sharp edges. I have a good friend who's a yoga teacher in New York and she says, 'Lean into the sharp edges.' I have this image of a very sharp metal point, and you're leaning into it as opposed to jamming into it. I just love that, so don't give up.

"One of the interesting things I find in observing, and through my own experiences as well, is that people go to a certain depth in their practice, they come up against the shadow aspect of it, and they say, 'Okay, this is boring or frustrating' or 'I don't like the feeling I'm getting from my practice.' So then they go, 'Well maybe Ashtanga is not for me,' so they go to Iyengar. They get a lot out of it. Then they come up to a certain point where they reapproach the shadow side to their practice. They go, 'Oh you know what? I'm frustrated and I'm bored and I'm angry. I'm going to try Bikram,' and there's this bouncing around, this search for the best yoga style."

Ted believes an experienced yoga teacher can help you navigate your sadhana journey. "Having a good teacher is going to give context to the experience, and the best teachers I've had are masters at that. They provide context to as much of the experience of the internal journey as possible. What we are encountering on this yogic path is hard, like really dark, and very challenging places mixed in with the inspiration or the beauty or the peace. There's a reason for it. The good teacher will guide you through those places, not as a therapist and not as a dictator but just as someone who's experienced it and who has a good ability to clarify what the unfolding will be. A great teacher would be a good storyteller, someone who has experienced their own challenges and hurts in the world and someone who has come out the other side with a sense of well-being or perspective and is able to not only illustrate but to verbalize."

However, Ted also advises using how you function in relationships and community as a reliable indicator of how well your practice works for you. "I don't subscribe to the guru model, and that may just be because I haven't met my guru yet. Thich Nhat Hanh said, 'It is possible that the next Buddha will not take the form of an individual. The next Buddha may take the form of a community.' When I first heard that, it was one of those moments when the whole universe just wobbled. How we interact is how our sadhana is created. So one of the things that we try to do within the Moksha context is continuously reinforce the idea of community, and that's our sadhana.

"I also think that the tendency we have to mythologize things and people and give them characteristics that aren't necessarily fair or true is epidemic in the guru model. Certainly, I believe deeply that there have been teachers in the past and possibly in the present that are worthy of that kind of elevation. But I also think that we need to continuously loop back to our present-moment experience and see how we're interacting and how we are in the world in relationship."

Ted has observed that partly through human nature, some yoga teachers are placed on pedestals by their students. However, if you put someone else on a pedestal, then where are you placing yourself? Ted values there being a quality of openness to sadhana, as he explains, "I have a bit of a pet peeve about the contemporary yoga world, and that is that there is this preciousness about it where people contract into an ideology and say, 'This is the way.' It's almost like a packaging and a marketing of their ideology. I think one of the great things about the potential for what we have in the yoga community is the ability to dissolve those things. I'm guilty of it with my involvement with Moksha, but what I'm hoping is that we never have a static sense of who we are, what we represent, and that the only constant is orienting ourselves toward peace. Jessica and I try really hard to keep knocking any pedestals out because the more people elevate you, the more they get a wrong idea of who you are. I don't know who I am day to day, and I want to keep it that way. I want to keep curious and interested and fascinated and grateful. If people try to create this projection of their own needs, then it is injurious not only to the practitioner but to the teacher as well."

This sense of openness is also incorporated into Moksha teacher training. "We have a strong impulse to not say Moksha yoga is the 'be all and end all.' Practice is a personal thing. You should go with what your phase of life is, your constitution, what you're looking for in your life, and suit your practice to that. In our teacher training, we have other styles of asana that we offer just so people don't get this idea that Moksha is this package that you have to live with. Every week we'll have a 'Freaky Friday'; we'll have a Yin class, an Anusara class, an Ashtanga class, a Restorative class, a Sivananda class to create this dialogue around what asana is and that it's not one thing."

Ultimately, just as an appreciation for life and love for the world we live in inadvertently led Ted to yoga, the same gratitude continues to fuel his practice. "I really am committed to the idea that my yoga practice isn't defined by asana. Certainly it's a component, but relative to how I want to move through the world, it's a combination of reverence and fascination. That's what keeps bringing me back to my sadhana: reverence for the ability of a seed to create a massive oak tree, reverence for the way that the universe unfolded, and if it were two degrees different at the inception of the Big Bang, then we wouldn't exist. Just the absolute mind-blowing beauty of how we are so privileged to be able to look out and interpret the universe and deeply witness the world around us. I find that beauty and fascination of existence to be what keeps me coming back to my devotion to practice. The practice of asana, the practice of sitting, the practice of contemplation; they all provide the stillness required to drop out of our conditional existence and perhaps just for a second to experience full peace in the world."

Chapter Twelve

Sat Dharam Kaur

Sat Dharam Kaur has practiced and taught Kundalini yoga for over thirty years. A practicing naturopathic doctor, Sat Dharam is also the author of *A Call to Women: The Healthy Breast Program and Workbook*, *The Complete Natural Medicine Guide to Breast Cancer*, and *The Complete Natural Medicine Guide to Women's Health*. She has also developed a yoga-based addiction recovery program and a breast cancer awareness and prevention program using the methods of Kundalini yoga.

From my first contact with Sat Dharam Kaur, she emanated a gentle sweetness in her presence. Similarly, it was a sweetness that captivated her and set her on a path of yoga from her very first exposure to sadhana. "The first time I was informed about sadhana, I was nineteen years old, and a friend of mine invited me to do a two-and-a-half-hour meditation with him at four in the morning. I had at the time been reading a little bit about yoga, and I was intrigued. I was very open, as I had no preconceptions at all. That was my first experience. It was an absolutely profound experience. I was hooked on the first try."

Since then, Sat Dharam Kaur has been devoted to Yogi Bhajan's 3HO organization's outlined practice of Kundalini yoga. To those of us not familiar with the practice, it might seem somewhat austere to discover that Sat Dharam gets up for a 4 a.m. practice every day (she doesn't go back to bed afterward), yet she describes those early years of practice with an air of liberating lightheartedness. "I was living in Toronto at the time, going to art school, and I just dived in, taking three yoga classes a day. I started teaching right off the bat because at that time there was not a teacher training. Yogi Bhajan just encouraged people to teach as soon as they learned something, so that's what I did. For a number of years early on, age nineteen to twenty-three, I was teaching my friends at the Ontario College of Art, so I was able to get paid to teach yoga at lunch hour. I was teaching at 7:30 in the morning and at 6:30 in the evening, and I was going to sadhana every morning at 4 a.m. At that time, Kundalini yoga was much more intense than it is now. Everything was sort of speeded up and involved very powerful breathing. It has mellowed out quite a lot since in general."

Sat Dharam and a friend helped each other to wake up in time for sadhana in those early years. "In Toronto there's an ashram which at the time was very disciplined. Anyone who lived there had to get up; it was expected, you had to get up for sadhana. I lived maybe a fifteen-minute bicycle ride away from the ashram. I would phone my friend who was also going to art school. We'd wake each other up, and we'd both ride our bikes and arrive at sadhana. She played the mandolin, and we had live music, and it was just totally awesome. There were usually thirty to forty people there, the room was packed, and you were lucky if you got a space. If you were late, there was no space. I did that for maybe two years, and then I moved into the ashram when I was twenty-one. There was simply an expectation that if you lived there, you did sadhana every day, which was very good for me because I was not particularly disciplined. Though I loved the yoga, the discipline, that setting, was a structure that suited me a lot. It's not hard for me to get up early and do sadhana because the tempo is there, the rhythm is set."

Sat Dharam Kaur was facilitating a weekend of classes in a town near my home when we arranged to meet during one of her breaks. She very graciously invited me to attend any portion of her scheduled weekend program. I chose an evening class, and, having never participated in a traditional early morning 3HO Kundalini-style sadhana, I opted to try that too. When I mentioned to a couple of my non-yoga-practicing friends what my plans were for the weekend, their reaction was typically along the lines of, "What? That's crazy!" However, when I arrived at the studio where the early morning sadhana was to be held, it felt magical.

A group of us gathered as the sun rose over the Rocky Mountains, to practice sadhana together. There was beautiful live music, singing, meditation, gentle lighting, and even home-baked treats afterward. It really was a very special way to start your day. However, as lovely as it sounds, Sat Dharam admits, there can be some challenges to getting up so early every day. "When I was going to art school, I would fall asleep in the afternoon in drawing class. I would have my hand on the paper, and my eyes would close, and I would nap for twenty minutes because I wasn't generally going to bed early enough. The challenge of living in this society where there is so much external stimulation and all the things that we have to do, whether as an art student or whether as a mother or a shopper or whatever it is, is that we're not living in a cave or a monastery where there are no other distractions. Even in the ashram in Toronto, everybody had their own life. Sometimes we ate together, we did sadhana together, we taught yoga classes, we attended yoga classes, but other than that you were expected to earn your own money, go to school, have a career. It wasn't a reclusive situation."

At times, Sat Dharam struggled to incorporate all of her daily responsibilities and a yoga practice into her day, as she explains, "One of the challenges of Kundalini yoga is that it is yoga for the householder. It's not meant to be a yoga of retreat, which was very difficult because there were no models, especially for women. I started Kundalini yoga when I was nineteen, and then I was in art school. Then I went to the University of Guelph and finished my bachelor of science degree. Then I went to naturopathic college and became a naturopathic doctor, but in my third year of naturopathic college I was pregnant, and in my fourth year I had a child. So to try to juggle all that and to know how to prioritize, how to do it all was very, very hard. There was this feeling of guilt if I wasn't up for sadhana. Eventually that went away, thankfully, and now I do it out of love."

As time passed, Sat Dharam started a family who also attended sadhana, and she found that just as her life changed so too the ashram continued to evolve. "In the Kundalini yoga tradition, we are encouraged to bring our children to sadhana, which I did for the most part. We would just pick them up and carry them upstairs at 4 a.m. I had three children while I lived in the ashram. I lived there for twenty years, and the ashram went through a lot of changes, from being very structured at the beginning to quite unstructured. It went through a rigid, structured, judgmental, fundamentalist period, and now it's quite loose. The building, the place, still exists, but now there is an eclectic variety of different spiritual traditions that live there. There is a Kundalini yoga sadhana that happens every day, but there are just two or three people who go and attend rather than thirty or forty as in the early days. It's healthy now because people are there because they truly take themselves there and believe in it, not because somebody is looking over their shoulder or they have to be there. It's been very interesting to see that evolution in one particular community, how sadhana has evolved over the years. That's kind of similar, I think, in all the 3HO communities, at least in North America, that it went through a trend of being very rigid, judgmental and hierarchical at the beginning to being more joyous, relaxed, and mature now."

Sat Dharam Kaur has also found in her yoga experience that an outlined structure often leads to an energizing, even healing, freedom. "I think it is very good to have a prescribed structure, at least initially, and that prescribed structure might be useful for a very long time. I still use the prescribed structure that Yogi Bhajan gave, and as time's gone on, I recognize the perfection and the beauty of that structure and the importance of all of its components more and more: it works. I think it is very easy if you don't have a prescribed structure to slip and slide, as though the more choice you have, sometimes the less discipline you have, until a person is mature enough and the sadhana is ingrained and they know what they need and they can do it for themselves. Yogi Bhajan said that if you do something for two and a half hours a day, which is what the sadhana is, one-tenth of your day, then the universal magnetic field holds that, almost as a structure, and reflects it back to you, so a lot of things change dramatically in your life. It's just that practice of two and a half hours. I believe that, and that's an incredible thing to experience."

For Sat Dharam, that structure comes from not only attending to her personal practice every day but also adhering to the traditional aspects of her sadhana, all serving to create a sense of specialness, of sacredness. "I think it's important to find or create a sacred space. So you wear your white clothes or your designated clothes for yoga that reaffirms, 'Okay, now I'm going to do my yoga practice.' Then you have your sheepskin or your yoga mat. You set it down so that there is a sense of place—this is where I do my yoga. In the Kundalini yoga tradition, we have mantras that we listen to. We have about a hundred different variations of the sadhana mantras, different music to go with it, and music is a structure. You put the tape on, and you have to go until it's finished, and so it holds you, it holds you in that space. Then we start with a prayer, the Japji prayer, that sets the intention of the mind. The next part is a kriya, which is about half an hour or forty minutes of yoga which might include a pranayama and a yoga set, and that yoga set could be the same every day. Often we pick something, and we do it for forty days or ninety days or 120 days to sort of dig into and gain the benefit of what that particular kriya is supposed to do, or you could vary it every day. Then you sit and open the heart with singing. You get into group consciousness with the singing. Then at the end, in many communities, you do a reading from the Sikh scriptures, and that becomes then the thought for the day, the orientation for the day, the personal message for the day. It's a gorgeous tradition, that whole piece, there's nothing missing. It's got all aspects of yoga in there. It's got the bhakti yoga, it's got the hatha yoga, it's got the pranayama, it's got the asana, it's got the devotion, it's got the wisdom, and it's all there in two and a half hours. It's just awesome."

In other traditions of yoga, I have experienced, and heard other people share their experience of, a connection to God or a divine energy or whatever greater power they feel they are connecting to or with. I have also read about it in the literature that describes and supports the study of yoga, but in the Kundalini tradition it seems that bhakti, even the use of the term, as well as its being an intention of a sadhana practice, is a little more "front and center." Sat Dharam agrees: "It also depends on what someone brings to a Kundalini practice. I think there are many people that could practice Kundalini yoga, and they don't have a whole lot of bhakti; maybe it'll develop over time, but we say with Kundalini yoga you need a balance of bhakti and shakti. The yoga creates a lot of shakti power, and unless there's the bhakti, it is imbalanced. The chanting and the reading of the scripture generates the bhakti, the postures are the shakti, and that's important because in this culture in North America, that's a little bit foreign: bhakti. I was raised Catholic, and I would say that I probably had some bhakti when I went to mass, but I didn't recognize it, yet when I go to India, if I go to the Golden Temple, oh my gosh, you are just overwhelmed with bhakti. It's so inspiring."

Many Kundalini yoga practitioners are not Sikh, just as many Sikhs do not practice yoga, but for Sat Dharam, the two traditions support her style of sadhana practice. "When I started doing yoga, I would say I was a pretty happy Catholic. I wouldn't say that I needed to go to church every Sunday, but I went to a Catholic grade school, I went to an all-girls Catholic high school, I was vice president, valedictorian, and all that stuff, and it suited me. I have no regrets about going to a Catholic school, but when I started to practice Kundalini yoga, it seemed like it was the wrong backdrop. Christianity didn't fit the experiences I was having or the worldview that went with the yoga. I wouldn't say that I denied Christianity, I just didn't have a devotional connection that fit, and the more I understood Sikhism I had no problem with it. It was when I was twenty-one that I took Sikh vows. There was a set of vows that you could take back then, and it was done almost, I wouldn't say impulsively, but my soul did it, and my ego wasn't quite ready for it.

"We have these big solstice celebrations, and one year I went to winter solstice in Florida, and there were probably a couple of hundred people there at the time. This was my first experience of solstice, and I literally thought I had arrived in heaven. I hadn't seen so much beauty and so much purity and so much grace in one spot ever before, and it totally blew me away. I determined at that time that I would wear a turban and become Sikh, and I knew that I had to become a Sikh officially or I wouldn't wear a turban. It's interesting because looking back I thought, 'How the heck did I do that?' because I actually fought it. I really didn't want it on an ego level, but it was a decision that my soul made. I just went along with it, and it literally did take me at least ten years to integrate it."

Though it took time to integrate the different aspects of her lifestyle and sadhana Sat Dharam persevered. As she explains, "I would be in Toronto trying to go to art school with a turban on. I had been one person a week before, and I came back wearing a turban. At that time it was very strange, and yoga was very strange, and so it was incredibly difficult. I felt like I was a split personality—one in the spiritual realm, one in the old realm—but once it all came together, it was magnificent. Now I'm pretty whole, and my spiritual identity has integrated very well with my personality, and my job and everything that I do, it's all of one piece. There's nothing that is not truthful for me in the things that I do in the world, and that's huge."

This sense of intuitive truth has worked to guide Sat Dharam, as she explains, "The other interesting thing about how my life has evolved is that everything that I am is kind of out of the box and self-created. I'm a naturopathic doctor. When I started in the naturopathic profession, there were fifteen people in my class, and we didn't know if it would last as a profession in Ontario. When I started wearing a turban, I had no idea if this organization would last. It's quite amazing. When I started writing *The Complete Natural Medicine Guide to Breast Cancer* and developed the Healthy Breast Program, I had no idea if it would fly or if there was a need for it, if there was an interest in it. I go forward with tentative intuition, and the universe answers back with gratitude and affirmation, and I say, 'Okay, I guess I'll continue with this project.' It's been a process of continual expansion and increasing confidence that even though I'm 'out of the box,' my intuition is correct and things that I'm called to do matter. I think it's really fun."

While spirituality has remained a significant aspect of sadhana and lifestyle for Sat Dharam Kaur, committing herself to a yoga path that she felt helped her to experience more love and devotion, she hasn't always received approval from others who have taken issue with life choices she has made. "I have two sisters. One sister disowned me; she became a fundamentalist Christian, and she said that I was going to go to hell. I really haven't spoken to her since, other than saying, 'Hello,' on the street every once in a while. My other sister initially tried to convince me that I was being brainwashed or had joined a cult, but now she's very respectful and admires what I've done and what I do, and she's often come to my yoga classes. My mother left me out of her will. My father eventually had Alzheimer's, so it didn't matter to him at that point, but initially he was very critical. None of my family came to my wedding, which is horrible. Most of my friends kind of dropped away, not necessarily because I was doing yoga but because I moved to Toronto, and I gathered a new group of friends who were artists or yogis, so my relationships changed.

"Basically I had to forge my own identity and trust who I was becoming and simply trust the process. It was very different back then because there wasn't a whole lot of cultural support at that time, in the late seventies, for wearing a turban or being a Kundalini yoga teacher, and I'm amazed that I stuck it out. Lots of people didn't, and I'm amazed that I found a profession that I could work at. I was thinking of becoming an art therapist after I finished art school because I knew I wanted to help people, and I loved art and I was very intuitive. I had my heart set on a specific university and I went there and had my interview. I had excellent letters of recommendation, I had excellent marks, I had everything I needed as prerequisites. When I called to ask why I wasn't accepted, they said, 'It's because of your dress, because you wear a turban.' That was the first time that I had felt absolute prejudice that affected me that directly, but interestingly enough, it was that rejection that then pushed me into naturopathic medicine, so it was good in the end."

While Sat Dharam believes that the prescribed 3HO Kundalini yoga sadhana practices (unless applied under special circumstances, such as pregnancy) are typically equally appropriate for men and women, where she does think there might be an imbalance is the way in which women are supported in regard to pursuing and practicing sadhana. This includes the teaching of spiritual knowledge and practices to the children who are also members of the spiritual community. As Sat Dharam explains, "When I lived in the ashram in Toronto, there was support for women and their families for a certain number of years so that other people might come and help me take my children upstairs to sadhana practice, that sort of thing. Ideally there should be a recognition that it's a community and children are everyone's responsibility; one woman can't raise three children, do sadhana, cook, clean, work, do all that on her own. It's best done as part of the community if it's going to be successful. I was busy trying to figure out how I was going to make a living, how I was going to put food on the table, how I was going to go shopping, how I was going to do my own practice, how I was going to study, how I was going to write my exams. What I would have loved is for other people to help me with my children's practice. My husband lived with me in the ashram, but was also busy earning a living. We found it difficult to do all that we needed to do as young parents as well as establish a daily practice with our children. That's the part where, if I could do over, I would want to see community support around helping the children maintain their practice and values because it's all about habit and the habits we are creating in ourselves and in our children. Yes, the children will model after us, and that's fantastic, but if we can create and instill in them these habits earlier on, they'll have them for life.

"I felt sometimes the pressure was so great. When I had my children, I took about a month off each time, and then I was back to working as a naturopath and doing my practice and teaching yoga and trying to write books. I was superwoman, and it was really hard. I did it, and I'm happy that I did it because it stretched me in all directions, but there's got to be an easier way, and that's community. That's why the community has got to be built around taking care of women and children so that the women can excel in their gifts and their strengths. There has to be absolute safety and trust; you don't want to entrust your children to someone who is not competent, but knowing there is a structure that holds the children and instills in them spiritual values and practices so that each generation is further ahead."

Despite the challenges that Sat Dharam experienced, reading before bed one evening, she discovered a sentiment that not only summarized her sadhana perspective but has also continued to inspire her practice through the years since. It was a line from a translation of the Sikh evening prayer called the Kirtan Sohila, and Sat Dharam describes her relationship with the prayer in the following way: "I don't read it every night before bed, but I was reading it one night, and the line was about the day is coming when I will meet my beloved. The idea is that you are going to get up and meet your beloved in the morning, and it hit me. It was like, 'Oh my gosh, if I say this every night, that tomorrow, I'm going to meet my beloved first thing in the morning when I get up, then I am going to meet my beloved.' It just put it in a whole new context that was so beautiful. I knew intellectually doing sadhana to be one with one's soul and to meet the beloved within was crucial for me rather than doing sadhana because you should or it's required or whatever it is. That's how I now approach it, and that's what gets me up: the meeting of the beloved."

That's a beautiful mind-set and motivation for lots of things really, but there are also more measurable outcomes of effort that can cultivate a more tangible impetus for a personal practice that Sat Dharam has applied to the structure of her sadhana at different times. "For ninety days I did a meditation practice called 'long chant' for two and a half hours each morning, which was something I had wanted to do for a long time. There are a few other techniques in Kundalini yoga that are two and a half hour practices that I would like to experience, so at some point I will choose to do something like that again, to really dive into one practice. But otherwise, I enjoy the prescription that we have, and I don't see that it would change unless, collectively, the group sadhana changes. When Yogi Bhajan was alive, he would change the sadhana every few years. Usually at summer solstice he'd say, 'Okay, now we're going to change the mantra, and we're going to sit in this position.' Japji was always what we read at the beginning, and then we always did half an hour to forty minutes of yoga, but the mantras changed, and basically the positions or mudras while you were doing the mantras changed over the years. In Kundalini, sadhana is recommended, whenever possible, to be done in a group. His teaching is that we go from individual consciousness to group consciousness to universal consciousness, and so, basically, if we are going to be having group consciousness, we need to be doing the same thing."

Although Sat Dharam does appreciate that people will find sadhana in their own way, she does recommend seeking out guidance. "To have guidance from an experienced teacher can help strengthen the quality of your meditation and to understand how that meditation process or chanting process could be made more potent through concentration. If one is going to spend sixty-two minutes chanting every day, then how are you doing it? Also, have the big overview earlier on of what it is that one is trying to do in terms of understanding how the Kundalini energy flows, understanding how the various nadis (energy pathways) work, understanding what kind of effort is required. Then having the inspiration or the reading material or the group support to really maintain that momentum and maybe finding a coach that can help you maintain your momentum; finding a yoga teacher that you admire. Do not be afraid to ask for support or help or a buddy or something that lifts you up and makes you accountable to yourself."

Sat Dharam also finds that music, especially performed live, can help support sadhana. "We have beautiful CDs, but there's nothing as fantastic as live music, someone coming and putting their devotion into it right in front of you because live music always raises the energy. In New Mexico, when we have the summer solstice, every day there are 2,000 people there for sadhana, and every day there is a different group of live musicians playing. The meditation starts at five in the morning with gorgeous music from different countries all over the world. That live music is really precious; we sing the same mantras, but people have developed their own musical variations of those mantras."

Mantra is a crucial element of traditional 3HO Kundalini sadhana practice, and it's believed by practitioners that the benefits of mantra work on many levels. As Sat Dharam explains, "Mantra itself, sound, creates structure and form, and the mantras are aligned with Totality and source and truth and beauty, and so if you are doing that, there is less of a chance that there will be a lot of darkness because you are re-creating, always. With meditation, you are breaking down the self, but you are also re-creating and attuning to the whole with mantra, and it's a little bit of protection, a safety net. The sound is continually creating this template, imprint, this structure, that the mind then attunes to unconsciously and consciously, and again that lifts us out of dark states, whether it's fear or anger or whatever."

Ultimately, Sat Dharam Kaur brings her own style of sweetness and compassion to the realization of sadhana, advising, "Pray, lean on the infinite, and ask God for help, or whoever it is that you pray to, for inspirational practice and be very, very patient, kind, and loving to yourself trying to maintain a discipline. Guilt doesn't work at all, and so try to maintain loving discipline every day."

Chapter Thirteen

Nischala Joy Devi

Nischala Joy Devi is the author of *The Secret Power of Yoga: A Woman's Guide to the Heart and Spirit of the Yoga Sutras* and *The Healing Path of Yoga*. She also created *The Abundant Well-Being* CD series and the award-winning audio book *The Secret Power of Yoga* and provides a free weekly sutra emailing service via her Abundant Well-Being website. A monastic disciple of Yogiraj Sri Swami Satchidananda, Nischala spent over twenty-five years receiving his direct teachings. She began to blend her yoga knowledge with her understanding and experience of working within the field of Western medicine. This then led Nischala to develop the yoga portion of The Dean Ornish Program for Reversing Heart Disease. Nischala continues to teach yoga students, yoga teachers, and yoga therapists internationally, including offering the Yoga of the Heart therapy certification program.

When you meet someone who knows or has studied with Nischala and her name comes up in conversation, the other person always starts smiling. Usually a realization that myself and the other person know Nischala results in the following statement or semblance thereof: "Don't you just *love* Nischala." That ultimately is Nischala's goal, not an egomaniacal drive for adoration but simply a spreading of awareness and practice of love, for the self, and for each other. This is brought about by Nischala encouraging her students to recognize the following: "Yoga is remembering who we are, why we're here and what we're here to do: to find our true nature. Yoga is a union which brings us to the self, a remembering."

When Nischala reflects back on her own experiences, her attraction to yoga was a pull toward remembering. "I think that's the way of grace because yoga is not something that I took on as an adult. Even as a young child, I went into meditation. I didn't know what it was called, but that's what I would do. I lost it for a couple of years, the teenage years, and then when I found it again in coming into yoga, I was so grateful. It's like finding a long-lost friend that you thought you lost contact with or will never see again. Every day, I feel grateful for it."

Nischala's recollections of there being a way of peace or of joy that could accompany you wherever you might be goes back to her memories of early childhood. "My mother sent me to day camp, which was not my thing. Being outdoors with bugs and all kinds of things; I hated that kind of thing. I remember getting on the camp bus early in the morning, and all the kids were shouting 'Yay! What are we going to do today?' I would just sit there quietly, close my eyes, and go into this trance like state. The bus would pull up to the camp, and I would go out and do whatever I had to and then do the same thing on the way home. It was a quiet time for me to just go within to this place of stillness where I could hear the commotion around me but I was totally still within."

Nischala's natural inclination for meditation as a child was confirmed for her when she was introduced to more formalized yoga practices as an adult. Although Nischala has practiced many tools of yoga over the years, it's the more subtle practices that continue to appeal to her. "I think it's a kind of a vector. It starts off where you choose a practice that helps enhance that part of you that is not developed, the spiritual part of you that is not developed, and then from there, it branches out to everything you do in your life. You have the formal practice, and then the spiritual practice so that everything you do in your life becomes sadhana for the experience of knowing who you are. I think people generally pick a sadhana that is the same as what they always do instead of picking something that is a bit different and that can expand them a little. I guess for me, the deeper practices were always the most important. I really didn't appreciate the physical practices as much as the deeper practices. It touched a place in me that I knew very well but got lost in the modern world, and it brought me back home to that place deep in my heart."

That being said, Nischala firmly believes that while the heart may lead the way, it is a balance of the heart, mind, and hand that evokes fulfillment and joy. "That's the greatness of yoga: finding the balance of the head, heart, and hand. Each one of them has something to contribute. Having time for study, having time to delve into self-inquiry, observing your life and what you want to do with it. Then having the devotional part, something that touches your heart; it could be chanting, it could be reading, it could be talking to someone. Then, of course, the hand is always in service. Service has to be a large part of your life, not just a small part. Not something like you go and give money on Sunday or read to someone for ten minutes a week, but something that really becomes your life so that everything you do becomes that service.

"I really feel that it has to be the three parts together. If it's not the head, heart, and hand, then we become imbalanced. If we're doing too much mental or we are doing too much heart, there's not that balance. A three-legged stool is a very stable stool. A one-legged or a two-legged stool doesn't have that stability. I've seen how people react when there's service in their life, and it gives a whole different meaning to life. Besides helping the person that you're serving, it's really helping you; you're the main one that it's helping. It's broadening your life and giving you something to look forward to. I try to have all those components in my life, and when I find that one is missing, I feel an imbalance."

Karma, that is, action or service, played a role in Nischala finding both this balance and being reintroduced to yoga. There was a time when the universe seemed to be telling her that she was on the wrong path, and the compassionate observations of another literally informed her of what she needed to do to find peace. "I had a car accident in Canada and we went over a cliff, and it wakes you up. I went back to the States, and I moved in with a friend who was starting to study yoga, and she encouraged me to go to a class. I did, and it was not really my style. It was much too physical for me. Then I moved to San Francisco and started working at a women's medical clinic, and it was extremely stressful. One night I went to the restaurant where I would go to eat every night because I was too tired to cook my own food. It was called Good Karma Café, and I was sitting next to this man who said to me, 'You look really stressed. Why don't you try some yoga?' He told me to go to Integral yoga. I did, and it was as if I was back on the bus on the way to camp. I just immediately tuned right into that same place again, and once I found it again, I didn't want to ever lose it."

Though Nischala felt an immediate affinity for yoga she appreciates that a personal yoga practice isn't always as instinctive for others. "In a way, that made teaching good and difficult at the same time because I didn't have a lot of the experience other people have with struggling to get a personal practice, so that was the bad part of it. The good part of it is I think other people could see my dedication and could be inspired by it. I couldn't really say, 'Oh, I had a hard time getting into it too.' I tried not to talk about it because I didn't want them to feel that I had difficulty or I didn't have difficulty and they do and they weren't as good as me. I tried to just tell them the incredible benefits of being inside and the joy that it brought."

A sense of gratefulness infuses Nischala's approach to sadhana, nullifying any sense of obligation, her instinctive tendency for practice being one of love. "When I lived in the ashram, we would meditate at five every morning, and I would always be there by 4:30 because I loved being in there before everybody. I liked what I called 'waking up the altar.' There were curtains around it, and I liked being the first one to open it. It was so regular that if I wasn't there, someone came looking for me. They knew I was really sick if I wasn't there. I had this incredible love for it. It was like having a lover for me, there was passion there. Some days I just sat chasing my mind around, but it didn't deter me because I knew what was coming: there was something there, it was just momentarily obscured. Everybody's been through difficult times. I've been through very difficult times, but I never abandoned sadhana because I knew that's what would get me through the difficult times and bring me to the real."

With such a focus on joy, love, and a connection to the divine through Nischala's approach to yoga, she does still appreciate the usefulness of asana but is wary of yoga being perceived as an exercise regimen. "A daily yoga practice doesn't have to be physical where physical exercise has to be physical. It's kind of obvious, but I think that's the problem: people think of yoga as physical. Most of the yoga practices are not physical, and that confusion leads them to think, 'Oh I can take a run instead of meditating,' and it's not the same. Meditation needs to be done in stillness. There's a mesmerizing effect of running, but it's a very different practice."

I sometimes wonder myself, in my own practice, if my being is telling me to cultivate a gentler practice some days or if I'm just simply being lazy. Am I practicing ahimsa, nonviolence, or, rather, compassion toward myself, or am I being overcome by inertia, by tamasic tendencies? Nischala believes it's more about santosha, a sense of contentment. "When we're content, when the sadhana is correct for us, and is right for us at that time because I think it changes, there's contentment, and a sattvic nature that comes forward. When the sadhana is not right, you may get more rajasic, you may get more agitated, and then it's not right.

"I was asked to do a five-day silent retreat on the East Coast of the United States and it was for a hatha yoga association. I said, 'You know, I really have doubts about this, whether they'll be able to sit.' They couldn't sit. They were so agitated because they did so much of this particular practice, and instead of feeling calm, the retreat did the opposite. It seems to me that there's a contentment, and it doesn't mean you have to be quiet. You can be in active contentment, but you're okay, you're happy with the way things are. There's a balance in your life and you feel it.

"Ahimsa versus tamas is totally different. My definition of ahimsa is having reverence and love for all, and that means you treat people in a certain way. Tamas, inertia, means you just don't care. There's nothing to get you moving; it's a very different experience. Ahimsa is as sattvic as you can get, as balanced as you can get, and you take action if you need to. Someone like Mahatma Gandhi was certainly with ahimsa, but he took action when necessary. Nelson Mandela, Mother Teresa, they all were people who needed to take action when they needed to, but when they didn't they were content, and they were finding reverence and love for all."

While Nischala firmly believes in the importance of sadhana and that it is a practice for her that has offered comfort and support throughout most of her life, she also believes yoga classes and yoga teachers offer guidance that can be key to developing our own personal sense of practice. "For most people it's inspiring, it's satsang. It's company with other people who are sharing your truth, the same truth. I think classes and personal practice are very different because in classes you have a teacher who hopefully inspires you and encourages you to do things that you may not want to do alone. The personal practice at home is a time to go deeper and maybe have that quiet time which you don't have in class.

"Guidance is very useful; people really need to have inspiration and to know that they're not alone. I get inspiration when I teach from the students, so it comes in different ways. When you're beginning, say, the first ten to fifteen years even of your practice, it's helpful to have a teacher, and even after that. Some of the teachers may not be in body, but they're still there. I lived with a master for twenty-five years, and it was invaluable for me because he didn't just teach me a few things, he taught me the whole gamut of how to live a yogic life. But now my teachers are less frequent because I probably don't need it. When I need it, they'll come more frequently. I feel I can call on a lot of teachers, in my inner guidance, for help."

When I traveled to meet with Nischala for our interview, I also attended one of her workshops, and the concept of fear in meditation came up for discussion within the group of yoga teachers present. I confessed to the group that there have been instances when I have been meditating when I have suddenly felt lost and startled that I didn't know where I was going and quickly retreated into more familiar meditation territory as it were. Being both my nature and perhaps human nature, to somewhat resist the unfamiliar and also to procrastinate about that which seems inevitable, I rationalize my decision with such thoughts as, "Well, I have three small children, pets, a home to look after, a marriage to nurture, my work. I'll have so much more time to meditate more thoroughly and with more dedication when I'm older. Maybe I'll save it for my retirement, like golfing, watercolors, and (if I'm honest) afternoon gin and tonics on a chaise longue too."

Another yoga teacher in the room suggested that perhaps it was more about a fear of a lack of control, a fear of completely letting go. Nischala compassionately nodded, smiled kindly, and explained, "The mind projects fears. There can be a fear of letting go, but it's only yourself. The knowledge, though, can be a risk. If while meditating you learn or remember something, it can lead to change. Some change is simple, but some can make it difficult to go on the same way if you haven't dealt with it outside of meditation, that's what the yamas are for. When you are going to meditate, always start with pranayama, it will balance your prana, energy, and fear is less likely to come into you. Fear of having to change can come with discovering more truth, but if you wait until you are older, you'll have lost the key and won't remember where you've put it. Samadhi is a gift; don't waste it by being afraid. Experiences like that are subtle. Don't whisk them away; accept them in gratitude."

One of the other yoga students attending the workshop confessed to me in break that she and her sister were talking only the day before about fear of where we might go in meditation and what we instinctively do to pull back or avoid it. She then told me that she was about to return to living in India (she was only home for a short break to meet her sister's new baby), where she normally abides either in ashrams or retreats to live in caves, to be able to withdraw from the world and dedicate herself to meditation. It was reassuring, albeit rather ironically, to realize that I wasn't alone being somewhat scared at times when I was alone.

Later during the same workshop, our quiet space was pierced by the sirens of an ambulance rushing by. Nischala paused and asked us all just to breathe for a minute and send loving thoughts to that person or more specifically to "someone who is scared right now." It might have been the patient in the back of the ambulance or someone waiting for it to arrive, but the conscious group effort to send peaceful thoughts and energy to someone we most likely don't know isn't scary in the least. If we can mindfully do it for them, surely we can do it for ourselves.

I explained to Nischala that after certain rather profound and unexpected meditation experiences, I sometimes have wished afterward that someone had been with me. Then I have realized that there is really only me to be with. Nischala's advice compassionately leads to the heart. "You have to go into your own heart. I go into my own heart, and it is as if I just curl up inside, and it holds me and sustains me. I think that we have to know where our heart is and how we can get into it, and I think that's what sadhana allows us to do. It's like curling up into someone's arms, but it's my own heart that does that because ultimately that's all we have anyway."

This compassion for ourselves and our sadhana also extends to being mindful of any stress we are creating in regard to our personal practice. Nischala advises being aware of whether your practice is meeting your level of stress or whether it is taking you away from stress. "Even a little bit makes a huge difference in your life. Even if you start out with five minutes a day, it makes a huge difference, and that difference will grow and change your whole life into something beautiful. The light within is always there, and if we're so busy that we can't pay attention to it, then often it remains behind a cloud. Sadhana is that which brings us into light. Then you can see the beauty in ourselves and the beauty in everyone."

Chapter Fourteen

Richard Miller

Founder, Executive Director, and President of the Integrative Restoration Institute, Richard Miller, PhD, is a psychologist, cofounder of the International Association of Yoga Therapists, and founding editor of *The Journal of the International Association of Yoga Therapists*, now known as the *International Journal of Yoga Therapy*. Richard developed the iRest protocol, a deep meditative yoga nidra-inspired practice that he shares and teaches via workshops, retreats, and teacher trainings. He is the author of *Yoga Nidra: A Meditative Practice for Deep Relaxation and Healing* and Richard has also developed the MP3 recordings of iRest practices *iRest at Ease*, *Resting in Stillness* and *Integrative Restoration*. Richard also facilitates research into the healing benefits of offering iRest to populations in diverse therapeutic settings, including within correctional facilities, with veterans, with people who are homeless, and with people living with post-traumatic stress disorder.

The Integrative Restoration Institute, which houses offices for iRest, is located in San Rafael, California. A few blocks away from the Institute which Richard founded is a beautiful sacred building, the Church of Saint Raphael, both the town and the church named after the archangel associated with healing. If you walk east of the church for a minute or two, you'll come upon the Integrative Restoration Institute which is also dedicated to helping people heal. The offices are close to the core of the town yet inconspicuously nestled in their surrounding nature, so unassuming that they could be easily overlooked. I was a few minutes early for my meeting with Richard, and so I sat in the office's wood-paneled waiting room. When Richard arrived he was welcoming and modest and he brought a lighthearted energy into the room. We chatted briefly with members of the iRest staff before retreating to his office for our meeting.

For a period in my childhood, I lived in a very small village in the midst of the English countryside. During this time, I attended confirmation lessons with the local vicar, and also being in the church choir, I met with the vicar's wife, a musician, for weekly singing lessons, both taking place at the village vicarage. Their children grown, the vicarage they inhabited was always quiet with a deep, historical peace, completely different to the kind of quiet that might occur in short bursts in my childhood home comprised of multiple siblings and their frequently visiting multiple friends. The vicarage space was framed and contained by deep, dark wood hundreds of years old that emanated a wise, oaky calm. Slow, quiet time was gently punctuated by the soft ticking of a grandfather clock that the vicar would adjust for me as I readied for home so I could experience what I very much considered the treat of hearing the hour chimes of the antique. It was otherworldly in a very peaceful way. At times since then, I have encountered spaces and places that emitted a similar energy and created a similar environment but perhaps none more so than Richard's office. The energy held within that space is very quiet, very still and very peaceful, a sacred space blessed with a composed calm.

A search for a deep connection to quiet peace is what originally drew Richard to yoga. "When I walked out after my first yoga class, I had a very deep experience of my interconnectedness with everything, and it felt to me that it was what I had been looking for for years. I remember as I was going home making a vow to myself that I would like to spend as much of my life as was necessary understanding this interconnectedness that yoga was evoking in me. I came upon a spontaneous sadhana vow without yet really understanding what I was leaping into, but it evoked in me a deep curiosity, wonder, and heartfelt joy that I had been looking for. I realized it was inside me, but I didn't have the tools at that time, so I wanted to find where I could feel supported in this new adventure."

Richard then began his yoga journey in earnest. "It was a very stimulating concept because it offered me a sense of home, structure, potential support, and community through which I could investigate. During that year, I began to read intensively and began to take up some preliminary sadhanas. I joined Paramahansa Yogananda's course and the following year met my first mentor, a woman from the Far East who had recently landed in the United States. She had been taught Buddhism and yoga as a child and had grown up in an Eastern community of meditation. Through talks with her, it continued to stimulate that sense of being on a path of self-discovery that grew into what I would now call my sadhana."

An awareness of sadhana began for Richard in 1970, realizing and revealing itself gradually. "I was taking classes at the Integral Yoga Institute in San Francisco and during that time I was reading into the field of yoga because I was taking the classes. I began to read into Satyananda's and Paramahansa Yogananda's writings and became aware of sadhana as a term and as an orientation to one's life."

Richard's development of sadhana continued, energized in part by joy. "I have come to understand one of the roots of the word of 'discipline' is actually 'love of learning.' I was excited about learning. I wouldn't say it took, in those early years, a willfulness. It was coming more out of joy and excitement and interest, curiosity, and also my own personal suffering that I was interested in bringing to an end: depression, isolation, and alienation kinds of feelings. I saw this sadhana path as a possibility for helping me resolve those inner conflicts."

This resulted in Richard's early twenties being filled with discovery. "I began to explore different paths in those first three years; 1970 to 1973. I was exploring Buddhism, I was exploring yoga, I was exploring Taoism, I was sitting in Zen retreats, and I was exploring Christianity with minor explorations into Sufism and the teachings of Gurdjieff. I was just seeing what was out there."

Richard founded the Integrative Restoration Institute in 2006, and the vision statement of this nonprofit organization asserts, "It is our vision to help people resolve their pain and suffering by rediscovering their essential wholeness and their interconnectedness with all of life." It was Richard's own distinct experiences of suffering that led him to seek out relief and that ultimately led to a personal practice and intentional application of yoga. "I would say from a very early age, nature was often more interesting to me than people. I would find myself in nature quite a bit alone, being quiet, walking, sitting, lying down. I had a natural affinity for silence. I also had some physical issues in childhood, especially some very severe migraine headaches that I had almost weekly. I learned that by lying down in a dark room with the lights off and my eyes closed, I could dive into the pain, and the pain would cease, and if I began thinking, the pain would come back. So I found myself lying in bed for sometimes four to six hours with my eyes closed, basically not thinking, and if I look back, I'd say my beginning experience in meditation was out of desperation."

Richard also experienced other happenings in his childhood that incited an inquiry into his sense of being. "I had experiences when I was young that left a deep impression upon me. One when I was about two and a half when, it feels now, looking back, my cognitive facilities came online. There was a moment where I perceived the world as separate from myself, and up until that time there was no sense of conscious separation. But in that moment, there was a conscious separation. When I look back at it now, it feels like that was the beginning of confusion, or wonderment.

"When I was thirteen, I had a spontaneous experience one night when I was lying down looking up at the sky and stars; a feeling of oneness that I would feel much later, but it was an extraordinary evening that left an incredible imprint in my psyche. Again I came to a moment where there was just a sense of oneness, no sense of separation; just an incredible sense of peace and joy, with no cognitive understanding, just the pure experience. Having a few experiences like that, and then going back into life where there was just a sense of confusion, stirred a deep inquiry in me of a deep sense of inner turmoil and a desire to bring it to an end, but I had no tools at my hand."

Richard did try exploring other alternate routes of finding answers to his anguish, but fortunately he was drawn toward more spiritual endeavors in his pursuit of both understanding and relief. "In my late teens, I got tangentially, not deeply, but tangentially, involved in taking LSD and mescaline and exploring peyote and had a number of experiences, but it didn't feel that it was a path for me. It opened up some doors, again I had some experiences of union, but it felt that they were state specific to the drugs. I couldn't maintain it during my daily life, so I didn't pursue that path. As I got involved in psychology, I began to use those tools, which helped to a certain degree, but I would say it was really when I began to meditate, to inquire into meditation and these deeper questions of 'Who am I?' and 'What is life?' that there began to be a resolution to the inner turmoil and suffering. Yoga really became an incredible doorway for me."

Richard's search for an end or alleviation to suffering in life also came to include striving to prevent suffering and unhappiness. "I began to gather around me people who were supportive, but the culture in 1972 and 1973 didn't really support yoga as a way of being very much. It was the end of the sixties, so there was some support, but I could feel I was walking a sword's edge. On one side was society which was saying, 'Become a banker, become a businessman,' and on the other side was this counterculture that was saying, 'Inquire, find out who you are first, and then see what you want to do,' and I landed in that camp."

This inquiry led to Richard making significant changes to the direction of his life. "In 1970, I actually had a job, a career pathway that would have ended in me being a branch manager for a large company which sold metal. I was training in it, and as I would sit at my desk, I would look at the people around me and have conversations with them and realized they were depressed, they were sad, they weren't fulfilled. I thought, 'Three years from now, I don't want to be sitting at this desk feeling unfulfilled.' When I quit and I went into the deeper studies of psychology and yoga, each of the people at my company who I'd become friends with took me out to lunch and congratulated me and said they wished that they were my age; that they would do the same but they had a mortgage, they had kids, and they felt they were trapped. That's exactly what I wanted to liberate myself from. I really felt called. It was a real calling, it wasn't a choice. I would say I had no choice. For my own well-being and sanity, I had to do what I had to do. That led sometimes to an extreme feeling of isolation and being alone, but there wasn't any hesitation in me. I knew what I had to do, even though I had no clue where I was going."

Although Richard took steps in what he felt was the right direction and explored different methods of relieving suffering, he began to feel torn; that he needed to commit himself more fully to the deeper study of, and application of himself to, one path. These feelings eventually led him to a conscious choice of dedication. "In 1973 and 1974, for me, there was a deep inquiry of psychology, yoga, psychology, yoga. My initial mentor had been teaching me in both realms, spirituality and psychology, and I started to feel too young as a psychologist or as a psychotherapist, and that I needed more maturing. The yoga offered me a possibility of doing something that I really loved. Out of that conflict, and in deep discussions with many people, I came to the conclusion to drop psychology and go full-time into yoga."

While Richard did commit to a full-time path of yoga, it did not come without challenges. "So in 1974, I opened a non-profit school of yoga that led me to walk away from my psychology practice and dedicate myself full time to yoga. I began in earnest to apply the teachings that I had begun to understand, and I also began coming to the ends of some paths. As I tread certain paths, initial excitement would blossom ultimately into a kind of feeling of a dead end which often left a feeling of despair and hopelessness at times."

Yet Richard's quest to relieve his suffering continued. "There came a moment where it felt like I was digging a lot of wells, and I made a decision to commit myself fully to the path of yoga. I dropped Buddhism, I began to drop my studies in Taoism. I really began to dig one well deeply, and I was involved in learning hatha yoga, pranayama, and the different meditation approaches of yoga. I was reading the *Upanishads*, the *Gita*, the different nondual texts. I was very immersed, and there were interesting moments where, for instance, I was doing four, five and sometimes six hours of hatha yoga a day, and I had, to a certain degree, mastered a lot of the different poses. I realized that ultimately while they made my body more relaxed and at ease, they hadn't ended my suffering, and I came to an end of hatha yoga. I took up more deeply the practice of pranayama and meditation, and I came to the conclusion with pranayama that it was relaxing my body and making me very subtly able to inquire, but it wasn't bringing an end to my suffering, so I came to the end of my pranayama. Then I just had meditation left. I was actually involved with a series of teachers and teachings, and each one I would go very deeply into. I studied with Bikram Choudhury, then Joel Kramer, and then with the Iyengar people and a man named Swami Bua and then the teachings of Krishnamacharya and Desikachar, and each one brought me along the path, but then, for me, ultimately I felt I came to the end of the teaching. It wasn't relieving my ultimate suffering."

Fortunately, for Richard, he met a teacher whose guidance helped him to bring an end to that sense of suffering. "In 1984, I met who would become my spiritual mentor, Jean Klein. When I first met Jean, he said, 'All of what you have done has brought you here; now all that you are doing will take you away from here.' So his suggestion was to stop doing. Stop searching, stop looking; just rest in your own being-ness. I took his advice, and I would say it was very good advice because it brought me ultimately back to myself. What's interesting is all along he was teaching hatha yoga and pranayama, so I never stopped my practices, I never stopped hatha yoga, I never stopped pranayama; I just realized there are limitations. They gave me good health, good relaxation, good resiliency, but they didn't bring an end to suffering but the path of meditation and self-inquiry helped bring me back truly to myself and brought an end to suffering: inner separation."

For Richard, the signs that he was at times traveling off course from where he needed to go on his sadhana journey were obvious and consciously recognized. At other times, his realizations were more symbolically conveyed. "There were lots of crises along the way. I was sitting on the floor of my yoga studio at one point just crying because I had come to the end of a teaching and I didn't know what to do. I was like, 'Okay, another teaching fails,' but it never stopped me from looking. I just said, 'Okay, what now?' I kept finding new teachers and new teachings, and one led me to the next to the next to the next. With one particular teaching I was involved in for a number of years, I felt like it was really taking me home. Then I had this dream where I was in a car with my teacher and the car was backing up, and when I woke up from the dream, I realized I was finished. I was backing out of the teaching, I was done with it."

Richard found his dreams often worked to help guide him as he searched for relief to his suffering. "I had dreams with other teachers when I wanted to really go more deeply into their teachings, and I would have these waking dreams with the teacher and the teacher would be saying, 'Stop, don't join me. Keep going.' So I kept going. I had different types of dreams: regular dreams, which were innocuous and didn't mean much to me. I would have teaching dreams where I would actually be with teachings and teachers I was studying with and felt like I was learning while I was dreaming. I had those dreams where the teacher or the teachings kept saying, 'Keep going.' Then I would have these other dreams where basically it would say, 'Stop; you're done.' Those times were very disconcerting because when the door would close, there wouldn't necessarily be another door that was opening right away, and so there were periods of despair or searching for what to do."

However guidance from a teacher helped to encourage Richard during these times. "My teacher, Jean, was very good. He basically helped me see, 'Don't follow me. Keep turning into yourself; the answer is in yourself,' because up until then I was still kind of looking outside. He really helped me come home."

Looking back, Richard feels like there was someone there with him all along, a companion helping to guide his way throughout that journey. It turns out that the companion was himself; Richard uses meditation to go back and connect with his younger self. As he explains, "I've gone back to every age I've been, and I've said to myself, 'It's okay, look who you turn out to be. You're going to go through some difficult times, and we're going to come out just fine. So I'm here walking with you even at times when you may feel alone and lost; it all turns out really good.' I feel now I was there for myself all the way along. There was something there, a force, guiding me all along, and it's been important to go back and reclaim that—just sitting quietly and taking an inner journey."

Richard views that practice of going back and revisiting his experiences as helping to complete his journey "home." "Now there is something I've come to understand as part of sadhana which is as we grow up, as I grew up, in my culture, my family, this society, and also as a human being, I see that I very naturally divided, separated, from other people, felt myself separate. I see that as a natural part of our evolutionary development as human beings. Our five senses and our mind create a sense of separation and distinction. Yet there's another: I call it the seventh sense. The sixth sense is the mind. The seventh sense is what knows interconnectedness, and I lost that thread in my early childhood. I think now I was trying to refind that thread, and yoga helped me relocate that thread that had just been covered over. In that moment in my early years until my mid-twenties, there was a feeling of division and an alienation from certain aspects of my being. Yoga brings an end to the game of hide-and-seek and we call, 'Olly, olly, in free,' and we start calling in all the disowned aspects of ourself, which I did. So part of going back to myself as a young child would be calling back all these different ways that I separated from myself, calling them back in to this sense of unification. Yoga for me was a homecoming, coming home to myself and then inviting all the disparate parts and aspects of myself back home too until there comes this incredible sense of healing."

One of my friends is a psychologist, and she often comments about how she finds it fascinating that we all do such different things with our lives, the different choices we all make in terms of what we eat, where we live, who we live with—we can all be just so different. I guess that might be what led her to study psychology. Somewhat similarly, I wonder what it is that makes those people we consider typically a little "different" different. They might excel at an activity or are fascinated by and study subjects to the nth degree, to the point where it seems like their behavior can't be explained simply by their choosing to apply themselves in a certain way, life circumstance, or opportunity. They really do seem to have come into this world with more unique expressions of a certain trait or ability. I wondered what it was through all those years of study and practice that compelled Richard to persist in searching for relief to suffering through yoga. Not that the yoga practice itself would be hellish, but without setting for himself a finite amount of time in which to find a definitive result to his quest, why didn't he give up and return to psychology or another spiritual tradition or choose to try something else entirely?

Richard explains, "I think it's just something innate. I'm very persistent and patient. I have tremendous endurance. It's innate to my character, and the practices helped bring it out and refine it. It's pretty difficult to tread these paths without some patience and persistence; that has to somehow arrive at some point I think, unless you're a lucky person who's just walking down the beach and it just hits you like a sledgehammer. For me I think it was innate curiosity and, again, suffering. I wanted to bring an end to it. I remember thinking when I read the Buddhist teachings, if I set aside that Buddha was born as a prince, he was just a human being. As a human being, he had the desire to bring an end to suffering, and he had brought it to an end. I thought, if he can do it, then it should be possible for me to do it, and if I can't do it, then probably nobody can because I felt myself to be as human as anybody else. I had this early-on understanding or orientation that I am going to do this, whatever it takes, or I'm going to die trying, and I was serious."

The morning I was on my way to meet Richard, I met a woman at an airport shuttle coach stop. Both of us had just arrived in San Francisco on separate flights, and while I was checking the schedule of the coach that I needed to catch, she walked up to check the board. She looked like a stereotypical lovely modern grandma with short, soft white hair, comfortable shoes, and a pastel-colored sweater embellished with flowers. Being the only people present at the coach stop, we began chatting as we waited. She was friendly, kind, and warm as she shared how she used to live in the Bay Area but had moved to a quieter place in the United States where she enjoyed the experience of "the full four seasons in the year," as she phrased it.

Our conversation soon turned, as these types of conversations typically do, to why we were visiting and where we were going. The lady I sat with informed me that she was in town because the court arraignment of the person who had killed her daughter-in-law and granddaughter was scheduled for that week. Her family members had been driving when a woman, distracted by texting, had driven into their vehicle, killing them both. How would you respond if a lovely person you just met sat next to you on a public bench told you that? I offered the standard though certainly sincere comments of sympathy and then asked her how she was feeling about the approaching week. "I *know* they're in heaven," she said, "so I'm okay with it." Although her life has been completely changed forever, I really did believe her—she knew that no matter what suffering might have been, or might occur, she *knew* it would be okay.

While Richard may have found the answer to suffering for himself through meditation and over years of practice has connected with a profound sense of peace, how does it feel to then observe the raw and unprocessed suffering or even trauma in others who are not at a place where the lady I met was, whatever the cause or manifestation of their illease or even pain? While Richard's daily work may be dedicated to helping other people to heal, what about the people who don't seek out help, whom he can't help or who even might seek out what they think is help only to intensify their pain?

Richard explains, "I feel the suffering of the world in other people, and yet I know underneath there is this thread of interconnectedness that they are not aware of. That gives me great solace and comfort because I know in the end it will be alright. I know where we all come from and where we are all going back to, so while another may be in deep suffering, I have a sense of where they are ultimately going to return to and that suffering will come to an end, even though it may be tremendous in the moment."

Although ultimately he found his own way back home, Richard is grateful for the many teachers who helped to point him in the right direction. "I think the guidance of a mentor who is walking ahead is really helpful. They're walking their truth, they aren't compromising; they are living examples of what I'm looking for. So Laura Cummings, Stephen Chang, Jean Klein, to me, were all living testimonials of the fruit realization of the practice. Each took me to a certain extent along the path, but Jean helped bring me really home. Support in terms of a teacher is really important. Is it absolutely necessary? No, because there is an inner teacher guiding our way always, and that inner teacher brings us to outer teachers. I have come to understand two types of teachers: ones who have given me means such as hatha yoga and breathing and meditation techniques; and teachers, in particular Jean and my early teacher Laura, who didn't give me so much teachings and things, they introduced me to the essence of who I am which no technique could bring me to.

"I've met enough people who have come to their own sense of peace and understanding without a teacher, but often, when I've talked to them, they ultimately needed teachers who helped them orient to what they had discovered because it was very confusing; it was disrupting all their beliefs and all their perspectives of the way of seeing reality. It was so disconcerting that when they found what I would call teachers or people around them who had that understanding and were oriented, it helped them orient. I think two in particular, Suzanne Segal and Bernadette Roberts, both when they woke up, it threw them both into crises. Whereas when they met people who helped them understand and orient to what they were experiencing, it helped them relax and settle in. So I think that teachers are extraordinarily important."

With such an immense explosion of yoga in Western culture in the recent past, I wonder how it might have been for Richard if he had been suddenly transplanted in time and found himself in North America, now aged twenty-two, setting off on a path of self-discovery with a quest to end suffering. "It would probably be just as trying and difficult; it might even be more confusing in some ways because we've sometimes thrown away the baby in the bathwater. I think historically Western culture isn't oriented toward gurus, but we are oriented toward mentoring. We have a history of apprenticing, and I think in the seventies, eighties, and nineties, there were so many gurus who took their students off the path because of their own misdeeds it's created kind of a crisis in the spiritual community of throwing away the gurus and looking for new models. I think the new model, at least for me, is that the guru for a westerner really isn't a guru; it is a mentor. It's someone who helps us apprentice into our self. I think it is a model better suited for us.

"If I were in my twenties now, there are tremendous teachers and teachings around that could help the pointing-out instruction happen perhaps a little bit more quickly, but I ultimately see it is still going to depend on the maturity of the student and their ability to grasp the teachings. I appreciate the tenacity of conditioning, and I appreciate the natural development of processes that I think are unfolding within each of us in an evolutionary way. You can't force yourself prematurely. We have to go through our own natural state of development, evolution, maturing. You can't rush the process. I think we can have mentors around us who perhaps help us stay closer to the path in not getting distracted, but even then, everybody has got to try their experiments. I'm a firm believer in the usefulness of the teacher but ultimately each person is finding their own way and has to do their own trial and error until they become convinced."

The sense of finding our own way and of learning our own lessons encourages us to welcome each opportunity as a chance to get that little bit closer to peace. However, Richard has found at times that he has had to carefully cultivate his sadhana path. "I had this image that came to me years ago, when I first discovered yoga, that it was like finding a very, very fine silken thread and if I pulled too hard on it, it would break and I would lose my way. Then I would refind that silk thread, and over years I would start to pull on it very gently through my practices. Pull on a thread, then a rope, and then a chain, and my practices helped me get hold of a very solid sense of the teachings. That said, I think it's easy to lose the thread when we're young and anxious to get on our way. The thread can break at times where we lose the scent, the fragrance that we're following, and then we have to stop. We may feel bewildered, but all of a sudden we begin to smell it again, pick up the fragrance, or find the thread, and then we start pulling again. Then out of our excitement, we pull too hard, and it breaks. I can see that's a maturity of learning, how to orient to the scent—a sense of unity and being-ness and interconnectedness. It's easy to get lost."

However, time spent searching is not time spent in vain. As Richard explains, "I never see karma as hindering. I always see it as another guiding force. I always felt like I was climbing a tree and I would go off on a branch and come to a dead end and go, 'Okay, come back. I'll go off here now. Okay come back.' Finally, we really get the scent of it, and we're not going off in the branches, we're just going straight up. Yet all those side paths have all taught me things that I can utilize in my own daily life and my work with people."

In his autobiography, Gandhi states, "The deeper the search in the mine of truth the richer the discovery of the gems buried there, in the shape of openings for an ever greater variety of service." When Richard decided to ask his now wife to marry him, he was basically living as a pauper in his yoga studio. His wife offered a compromise that led Richard to a new way of incorporating yoga into his life. "She said, 'Let's live together,' and I said, 'I'm done with living together, let's get married.' She said, 'Well, okay. You get a job.' So I went for a long walk in the hills of Fairfax, and I had like a bolt of lightning go through my body, and I actually heard this voice say to me, 'Psychotherapy.' A week later, I had an office, I had a practice going, I was seeing clients, and I started my income stream doing my practice of psychology where my practice of yoga was fully integrated. What I had originally perceived as a conflict in 1973 had resolved itself, and the two came together. I was practicing yoga and psychotherapy with people and really interweaving all of my teachings and training in yoga with my psycho-therapy."

Richard found that this merging of skills and knowledge helped realize his sadhana in a day-to-day way. "My desire was, 'How do I integrate this fully into my daily life?' If yoga is really truly a path for a westerner, then I should be able to hold a job, be married, have children, live a householder's life, and have it fully integrated with no conflict. I feel like that has been a big part of my sadhana, the integration of living. I actually had two teachers who both told me that if I was to succeed along the path of sadhana, I would need to leave my wife, leave my job, and leave my children. Both those teachers I left, feeling that that may have been true for them growing up in the East in their culture, but if this path of yoga is really truly made for a westerner, then we've got to find our own way of integrating it into daily life. Not as a monastic tradition but as grounded in a householder's moment-to-moment life."

Richard did come to integrate his sadhana within his more western style life. As he explains, "There were conflicts along the way. I had some deep challenges that I had to learn how to navigate, and my wife and I learnt how to navigate. It is a challenge to integrate, especially when your spouse doesn't necessarily understand the path you're treading. I think she didn't for many years, and it was confusing. Now she does, and it's fully integrated into our life and our relationship, but I see it as very challenging for couples when one has such a deep turning inward and the other doesn't understand it. It's a very challenging aspect of the path."

In a similar way, early on in Richard's life, his parents didn't quite understand their son's choices, but in the end they all came to be at peace with their relationship and with each other. "Neither of my parents were religious. I remember as a young child asking them if we could go to church because I was brought up Protestant. They weren't interested, but they took me to a church, I think more to convince me not to go. They wanted me to go to boarding school, and the boarding school I chose was St. George's, which had church every day and twice on Sunday. I loved being inside churches and cathedrals because they just felt so quiet."

This difference in perspective continued as Richard became an adult, albeit respectfully so. "I wouldn't say there was ever a conflict. My mom once wrote me a letter when I had sent her a bunch of yoga books and things that I was studying at the time. She returned them to me unread in a box and said, 'You must understand Richard, we're cats and you're a dog, and cats and dogs just don't understand each other.' I figured, 'Okay, they're cats and I'm a dog, they don't understand me, but I'm going to write them letters anyway just telling them what I'm doing.' So I wrote my dad this long, long letter about the practices that I was doing and the experiences I was having. He wrote me back this letter, and he said, 'That was the most beautiful letter I have ever been sent or read. I didn't understand a word you said, but that you would send it was lovely.' I would write them letters saying, 'I'm really thankful that you were my parents; I appreciate all that you did for me.' I would thank them, but I knew that they didn't have a clue. It just wasn't in their bailiwick, and I was from outer space."

On reflection, Richard feels that this sense of feeling different also helped to incite his journey of self-discovery. "I was a stranger in a strange land growing up. That was, I think, part of my suffering. I wasn't in an environment where I felt understood, seen, heard. I couldn't talk about what was going on inside of me, so I learned to be quiet. I think that stood me in good stead in that I learned to be quiet, and it stood me in bad stead because it opened up a whole sense of separation. Why am I so strange? Why am I so weird?

"I would try to join groups of boys and girls who were having discussions and they would be talking about this or that, and I had no interest. I found that in high school. I found that in college. I would get into the dorms and join groups that were having conversations at night, and it just never made sense to me because to me they weren't talking about what was real. They weren't talking about silence or themselves. They were talking about baseball, football, cars, and that just held no interest for me, and so that made me feel even stranger. I remember thinking to myself, 'I can't do the social thing. I don't know how to socialize.' I learned how to do it, but parties still don't hold much interest for me. I'm not interested in talking about things. I can do it for a little while, but I'm more interested in the inner life and what's really going on with a person. Who are they? What makes their life work or not work? What are their emotions like? Do they love themselves?"

Richard's life choices and way of being were reflected back positively through his sadhana despite how he might have been questioned about his choices over the years by others. "Sadhana means to me a life path, a way of living one's life. I still have old friends who come up to me and say, 'Are you still doing that nondual yoga thing?' and I say, 'Of course, it's the way I live my life.' I've also come to understand it as offering delicious tools for inquiring and supporting that way of being; it's tools, it's path and it's the fruition too. I found a sense of peace and harmony that has brought me to, on one level, not looking for anything anymore. That initial yearning has been satisfied, and now there is a whole other movement that has sprouted out of that path of sadhana. I think of it as a path, a means, the goal itself."

Sadhana has also brought other benefits to Richard's life, providing not only a coming home to himself but also a deeper connection to others. "Sadhana entails an interesting paradox between an inner calling where one walks the path by oneself, yet I have found an incredible community of like-minded brethren, and we're all walking the path together. That's been a wonderful discovery."

Richard also feels that there's a common link among the teachings he's been exposed to during his sadhana journey. "I would say every great book I've ever read, every great teaching I've ever received, every great teacher I have ever been with have always said only one thing: 'Be.' The simple sense of being is always with us, but we ignore it for another thought or another feeling or something else we think is more complex but to settle into the simple sense of being so that it awakens as a constant companion all day long; I see that it forms a trustworthy anchor so that when we begin to move away from our self, stray from the path, it helps call us back. We can feel, in comparison to the peace of being, the disharmony when we start to go away from our self. That contrast between the deep peace of being, and the disharmony of dividing from ourself allows us to see the error that we're engaging in and come back. Ultimately as we fall into being, we find a sense of harmony that's always been waiting for us."

While Richard's dedication to sadhana has brought joy, it is ultimately his commitment and inquiry into self through meditation that has brought a conscious alleviation to his suffering. "Meditation opened me to the understanding of how my mind works and to not get caught up in thinking. It helped me understand how my emotions work and to not get caught up in reactions. It helped me investigate and see my conditioning in a way to break free of my conditioning. It helped me understand the functioning of my body and my senses so as to not get caught up in them. Being free from body, senses, and mind—that allowed my free attention to turn back into, and inquire as to, who I am as awareness. To me, meditation is a feeling, inquiry, and as I felt into this quality of pure awareness, pure being, it kept liberating me into a sense of peace and harmony. Also meditation helped me understand myself as a human being, as an animal. It helped free me from taking things personally, both what was happening in me and happening in other people."

Richard's development of meditation came to include yoga nidra, which greatly impacted his practice, as he explains, "Yoga nidra was a very important doorway. I came to the path of yoga nidra in 1970, and I slowly evolved into it and it gave me an exquisite set of practices that helped me understand my body, mind, senses, emotions, and thoughts. It helped me heal through them and to a certain extent, get free of conditioning and re-activities. That then allowed my attention to be more and more free. That free attention now got to turn back into being and pure awareness, and the teachings that I really have loved all along from my very early days until now have all been direct pointers back to that basic ground of being and letting go of techniques. I find meditation has evolved from the discipline of sitting to a love of just sitting and just resting and abiding in being. I still do the hatha yoga, I still do the breathing, because they help calm the mind and keep the body healthy and resilient, but I love how they help support and bring me to an easy sense of being which is ultimately independent of technique."

While Richard's life is now deeply infused with a practice of meditation, he remembers his early attempts at meditation with a fondness. "When I took meditation on as a discipline, I remember playing with it and I would decide things like, 'Okay, I'll meditate for five minutes. If at the end of five minutes I don't want to meditate anymore, I'll stop.' But what I came to realize is five minutes in, I enjoyed myself."

Richard now considers meditation, like sadhana, to be an inherent part of every day. "Meditation has now become a twenty-four-hour affair. Yoga nidra has helped me bring the meditation into deep sleep, so it feels like meditation has become a continuity of all day long and all night long, and has interwoven into my relationships and into my work. I love the special time of sitting, but I must admit it has become just the fabric of my life. Sadhana has become the way I live my life. Meditation has become the way I live my life."

That isn't to say that Richard doesn't still attend to other aspects of his nature that require upkeep or nurturing. "I can't imagine until I get really old giving up my hatha yoga and my pranayama. It's like flossing and brushing my teeth; it's just something I do every day. Do I love brushing my teeth? No. Do I love flossing my teeth? Not really. Do I love doing hatha yoga? Not really. Do I love doing pranayama? Not really. But I know that they work, and when I get into doing them, I enjoy them."

Richard's sadhana now includes helping other people find their own way home. "Paradoxically, we're not going to find what we're looking for in yoga. People don't often understand me when I say it, but I think yoga works because it's designed to fail. It's designed to exhaust our looking outside for our source of happiness. It turns us slowly into ourself and away from the very techniques that it has offered us and that we come to the end of. We realize they didn't truly give us our freedom, but in exhausting them, yoga supports us into that deep inner inquiry, where we discover this deep innate happiness that's always been waiting for us but we've been looking for it somewhere else. It's been patiently waiting for us inside."

Richard tries to exemplify that sense of being to his students in the following way. "I ask my students the first time I'm with them, 'Do you know the sense of being when you're just between two doings and you're just being?' and everybody says, 'Yes.' Then I ask them, 'So when you're just being, where do you feel you are physically? Find yourself; where's your center, and where's your periphery?' Everyone comes to their own wording of it, but basically they come to this feeling of, 'I feel like a field of spacious openness, everywhere and nowhere in particular.' Then I ask them, 'When you're just being, is there any sense of time?' and they say, 'No, because the mind slows down. It's just timeless.' Then I ask them, 'Does being need anything that would make it any more perfect?' and they all say, 'No.' I ask 'Do you need to know anything that would make being any more perfect than it already is?' They say, 'No,' and I say, 'Do you need to do anything?' They say, 'Well I'd like to be more, but no, I don't need to do anything to be.' I say, 'Great, so now you've found you're spacious, timeless, perfection, completeness, and wholeness. Let's just rest here.' "

Epilogue

The night before I did my first interview for this book, I had a strange dream—strange not so much for its content but for its environment. I don't usually notice weather in my dreams; the dream just *occurs*. In this particular dream, it was evening, and it was raining heavily. I could feel the raindrops; I could see them, I could smell them, and I could hear them fall on the streets, windows, and roofs. It definitely wasn't actually raining outside that night (I live in a very dry climate), so there wasn't any kind of external world reality blurring into subconscious dreaming. The dream hung about my thoughts the following morning with me repeatedly summing up, "Wow, it was really weird, though, to keep noticing the rain and for it to even be raining in my dream." I googled it. I found that to dream of rain and to hear it drumming on a roof means you are inline for some kind of spiritual awakening. My reaction was along the lines of, "Hmm, that's a funny coincidence."

I met with my initial interviewee later that morning, a yogini friend who agreed to do a test-run question-and-answer session with me. Halfway through the meeting, she said something so touchingly profound that I started to cry. Typically, I'm not much of a crier, but we stopped our discussion, and I told her about the dream and how what she had said affected me. Both of our eyes welled up in the bustling coffee shop for a moment or two, and then we started to laugh. "How am I ever going to do these interviews if I just start blubbing every time someone might say something profound or touching or wonderful? They'll think I'm a complete nut case!" I asked. Her advice, as always, was honest and good: "You can show that you're a real person with real emotions, it might endear you to them a little more, it's humanizing."

So did I sob and blubber through every sadhana-focused conversation? No. Was each one wonderfully enlightening in its own way? Did I feel privileged to hear these unique tales of experience and viewpoint? Absolutely, every time.

I tried my very best to go into these interviews with no expectations, to be open to the information offered, yet during every conversation at some point, I was thrown or completely blown away by a message or sentiment being conveyed. For as much as I felt honored to be privy to the stories shared, I was also at times overwhelmed by the responsibility of recording and retelling those same accounts of decades of practice and experience. Put together, the people included in this book have the experience of centuries of yoga practice to share. I strived to honor that responsibility as best I could when putting together this manuscript and decided early on not to translate what they had to say at all; their stories were best told in their own words. The response I received from all of those included and from other teachers and practitioners, yogis, and yoginis who are not included in this book was overwhelmingly positive, and I will always be grateful for that support and trust.

I did find it interesting that for most of those included in the book, the age of eighteen or nineteen or even early twenties seemed to bring about a strong urge to explore philosophies, experiences, knowledge, and spirituality typically outside, in the pre-yoga boom past at least, of a westernized norm. In our North American society, often this is the age when children typically do or start to think about leaving home and I wonder if we do a slight disservice to our own younger generations in perhaps not offering more spiritual guidance in whatever form that might take as our children set off to make their own way in the world.

I have a furrowed brow, and I can over-think things to the point of once wondering aloud, "I think I might be indecisive. What do you think?" with no awareness of irony and, as usual, all seriousness. During the process of writing *Sharing Sadhana*, I've learned to lighten up a little more (not entirely, as I am who I am), but personally I don't believe in the labels of introvert and extrovert. I believe we live on a continually fluctuating scale of behavior, thought, emotion, and so on, and it is affected by our environment, company, food intake, sleep deprivation, what we have been taking part in or exposed to in the recent and not so recent past, and so on. The information I was privy to through the contained interviews has led me to live with a little more "lightness" and for those fluctuations in mood, behavior, thought, and so on to be a little less uncontrolled and to affect me unawares, just as the second Yoga Sutra tells us.

In writing this book, I'm not being precocious or deceitful or promising that it is a direct response to the conversations I took part in, or that it might have the same effect on anyone else, but, caveats aside, my physical body released a little; my practice physically opened as I spiritually opened.

Sounds cheesy, I agree, but it's true. It really did, honestly, not least of all because I cared *less*. In realizing and reaffirming that I know what is best for me, that I could let go of certain demands and expectations, everything softened, everything began to let go.

While traveling for the purpose of this book, I usually participated in yoga classes with the teachers whom I met in person to interview. It can be a little humbling exposing yourself in that way, and I certainly had a humbling experience. In one class, which was very physical but very knowledgably and compassionately taught, I was attempting to get into headstand and, unlike every other time I now do it both in class and at home, I came crashing down to the ground. When I say "crashing," I mean I fell in a very noisy and messy heap and almost took other people down with me: I crashed. I found it funny at the time. "Typical," I thought, "I couldn't possibly seem graceful and experienced right now—ugh. Take that, ego." Less than twenty-four hours later, I was in a completely different city taking part in a class with another teacher I was due to interview later that day. It was one of those classes where you feel like you are, as Doug Swenson puts it, "in the zone." After class, a teacher who had been adjusting and assisting during class approached me, introduced herself, and said, "You have a very beautiful practice." No one has ever said that to me either before or since and likely never will again. My point is that all that really matters in terms of my practice is how it makes me feel; some days I'll very ineptly fall and a roomful of people witness it, and some days I'll be complimented, but it's still me.

More than anything, I found the information shared by those interviewed liberating. As mentioned in the chapter focusing on Erich Schiffmann, I don't think it is a coincidence that the one term I heard over and over was "you know." It can be a flippant addition to conversation that is expressed in the pauses, or even to create those pauses; it may be hidden in between sentiments or in between thoughts, but it is true. In my yoga student experience so far, the people I have considered the best yoga teachers I've been exposed to have shown me that I already know what I need to know. They have shined a light on that knowledge or exemplified how a yoga practice or yoga "tools" can be used to enable or support me in accessing that wisdom and understanding, and shown me how I can use my own internal compass to guide myself along a yoga path, as Richard Miller explains, to coming "home."

In listening to the stories contained in this book, I found a comfort in knowing that so many people have chosen the route of yoga before me and are willing to share their experience of what decades of practice can bring. I equate it with falling asleep in my bedroom as a child listening to the soft voices of my parents as they talked in the next room—there's a murmur of companionship and competence in the dark we can all sometimes feel. Luckily, there are many yoga books to read that can help guide us on our sadhana path. I hope the stories contained in this book can help shine a little light for you on your way. Namaste.

Bibliography

Tagore, Rabindranath, *Sadhana: The Realization of Life*, Filiquarian Publishing LLC. edition, 2006.

Articles

Dubrovsky, Anna, "Radical Healing: Yoga With Gary Kraftsow," *Yoga International* Magazine   http://www.himalayaninstitute.org/yoga-international-magazine/inspiration-articles/radical-healing-yoga-with-gary-kraftsow

Press Releases/Websites

"Yoga Journal Releases 2008 'Yoga in America' Market Study," *Yoga Journal*, press release, http://www.yogajournal.com/advertise/press_releases/10, February 26, 2008.

"A Growing Profession: 70,000 Yoga Teachers Estimated by NAMASTA," the North American Studio Alliance, April 12, 2005.http://www.namasta.com/pressresources.php

http://www.namasta.com/pressresources.php

Resources

- Nischala Joy Devi: http://www.abundantwellbeing.com
- Sat Dharam Kaur: http://www.kundaliniyogatraining.com/
- Ted Grand: http://mokshayoga.ca
- Paul Grilley: http://www.paulgrilley.com
- Susi Hately: http://www.functionalsynergy.com
- Leslie Kaminoff: http://www.breathingproject.org and http://www.yogaanatomy.org
- Gary Kraftsow: http://www.viniyoga.com
- Molly Lannon Kenny: http://samaryacenter.org and http://mollylannon-kenny.com
- Sarahjoy Marsh: http://yogajoy.net, www.living-yoga.org and http://www.amritasanctuary.com
- Richard Miller: http://www.irest.us
- Wade Imre Morissette: http://www.wadeimremorissette.com
- Robin Rothenberg: http://www.essentialyogatherapy.com
- Erich Schiffmann: www.freedomstyleyoga.com
- Doug Swenson: http://www.sadhanayogachi.com

About the Author

Victoria Bailey is a yoga student, a yoga teacher and certified yoga therapist. Victoria is also a freelance writer and lives and practices yoga in Calgary, Canada.